PRACTICING PSYCHODYNAMIC THERAPY

Also Available

Psychodynamic Therapy:
A Guide to Evidence-Based Practice
Richard F. Summers and Jacques P. Barber

The Therapeutic Alliance:
An Evidence-Based Approach to Practice
J. Christopher Muran and Jacques P. Barber, Editors

PRACTICING PSYCHODYNAMIC THERAPY

A Casebook

Edited by

RICHARD F. SUMMERS
JACQUES P. BARBER

THE GUILFORD PRESS
New York   London

© 2015 The Guilford Press
A Division of Guilford Publications, Inc.
370 Seventh Avenue, Suite 1200, New York, NY 10001
www.guilford.com

Printed in the United States of America

This book is printed on acid-free paper.

Last digit is print number: 9   8   7   6   5   4   3   2

The authors have checked with sources believed to be reliable in their
efforts to provide information that is complete and generally in accord
with the standards of practice that are accepted at the time of publication.
However, in view of the possibility of human error or changes in behavioral,
mental health, or medical sciences, neither the authors, nor the editors and
publisher, nor any other party who has been involved in the preparation or
publication of this work warrants that the information contained herein is
in every respect accurate or complete, and they are not responsible for any
errors or omissions or the results obtained from the use of such information.
Readers are encouraged to confirm the information contained in this book
with other sources.

Library of Congress Cataloging-in-Publication Data

Practicing psychodynamic therapy : a casebook / edited by Richard F.
Summers, Jacques P. Barber.
     pages cm
Includes bibliographical references and index.
ISBN 978-1-4625-1718-3 (hardback)
ISBN 978-1-4625-2803-5 (paperback)
1. Psychodynamic psychotherapy—Case studies.   2. Psychotherapy—
Practice.   I. Summers, Richard F.   II. Barber, Jacques P., 1954–
RC489.P72P73 2015
616.89′14—dc23

                                                    2014025246

For my father, Robert Summers,
and my father-in-law, Arnold Bloom
—R. F. S.

For my mother, Lucienne (Sarah) Barber,
and my grandchildren, Luke and Jonah
—J. P. B.

ABOUT THE EDITORS

Richard F. Summers, MD, ABPN, is Clinical Professor and Co-Director of Residency Training in the Department of Psychiatry at the Perelman School of Medicine of the University of Pennsylvania. He has written extensively on psychodynamic therapy, the therapeutic alliance, psychodynamic formulation, psychiatric education, and positive psychology. Dr. Summers is the recipient of numerous national and local teaching awards, serves as Chair of the American Psychiatric Association Council on Medical Education and Lifelong Learning, and is a member of the Psychiatry Review Committee of the Accreditation Council for Graduate Medical Education. Past president of the American Association of Directors of Psychiatry Residency Training, he maintains an active clinical practice. Dr. Summers coauthored, with Jacques P. Barber, *Psychodynamic Therapy: A Guide to Evidence-Based Practice,* a widely used resource for seasoned practitioners as well as psychiatry, psychology, and social work students.

Jacques P. Barber, PhD, ABPP, is Professor and Dean of the Derner Institute of Advanced Psychological Studies at Adelphi University; Emeritus Professor of Psychology in the Department of Psychiatry and in the Psychology Graduate Group at the University of Pennsylvania, where he was formerly Associate Director of the Center for Psychotherapy Research; Adjunct Professor of Psychiatry at New York University School of Medicine; and Adjunct Professor at the School of Psychology and Counseling of the University of Queensland, Brisbane, Australia. His research focuses on the outcome and process of psychodynamic and cognitive therapies for depression, panic disorder, postttraumatic stress disorder, substance dependence, and personality disorders. A past president of the Society for Psychotherapy Research, Dr. Barber has published more than 180 papers, chapters, and books in the field of psychotherapy and personality. Among his more recent books are *Echoes of the Trauma: Relationship Themes and Emotions in the Narratives of the Children of Holocaust Survivors*, coauthored with Hadas Wiseman; *Psychodynamic Therapy: A Guide to Evidence-Based Practice*, coauthored with Richard F. Summers; and *The Therapeutic Alliance: An Evidence-Based Guide to Practice*, coedited with J. Christopher Muran.

CONTRIBUTORS

Jacques P. Barber, PhD, ABPP, Dean and Professor, Derner Institute of
Advanced Psychological Studies, Adelphi University, Garden City,
New York

Karla Campanella, MD, Psychiatrist in private practice; Psychiatrist,
Philhaven Behavioral Health and Cornerstone Family Health Associates;
Consulting Psychiatrist, Physicians Alliance Limited, Lancaster,
Pennsylvania

Samuel J. Collier, MD, Assistant Professor, Department of Psychiatry,
University of Texas Southwestern Medical Center at Austin;
Seton Family of Hospitals, Austin, Texas

C. Pace Duckett, MD, Psychiatrist in private practice, Bryn Mawr,
Pennsylvania; Clinical Associate, Department of Psychiatry,
Perelman School of Medicine, University of Pennsylvania,
Philadelphia, Pennsylvania

Lauren J. Elliott, MD, Psychiatrist, Psych Associates of Maryland,
Towson, Maryland

Patricia Harney, PhD, Associate Director of Psychology and Psychology
Training and Director of Psychology Internship Training, Cambridge
Health Alliance/Harvard Medical School, Cambridge, Massachusetts

Kimberlyn Leary, PhD, MPA, Chief Psychologist, Cambridge Health Alliance,
and Associate Professor of Psychology in Psychiatry, Harvard Medical
School, Cambridge, Massachusetts

Kevin McCarthy, PhD, Assistant Professor, Chestnut Hill College,
and Research Associate, Department of Psychology, University
of Pennsylvania, Philadelphia, Pennsylvania

Margot Montgomery O'Donnell, MD, Clinical Associate, Department of Psychiatry, Perelman School of Medicine, University of Pennsylvania, Philadelphia, Pennsylvania

Bianca Previdi, MD, Clinical Associate, Department of Psychiatry, Perelman School of Medicine, University of Pennsylvania, Philadelphia, Pennsylvania

Dana A. Satir, PhD, Clinical Assistant Professor, Department of Counseling Psychology, University of Denver, Denver, Colorado

Robert Schweitzer, PhD, Associate Professor, School of Psychology and Counselling, Queensland University of Technology, Queensland, Australia

Dhwani Shah, MD, Clinical Associate, Department of Psychiatry, Perelman School of Medicine, University of Pennsylvania, Philadelphia, Pennsylvania; Staff Psychiatrist, Counseling and Psychological Services, Princeton University, Princeton, New Jersey

Brian A. Sharpless, PhD, Assistant Professor of Psychology and Director, Psychology Clinic, Washington State University, Pullman, Washington

Richard F. Summers, MD, Clinical Professor of Psychiatry and Co-Director of Residency Training, Department of Psychiatry, Perelman School of Medicine, University of Pennsylvania, Philadelphia, Pennsylvania

Holly Valerio, MD, Clinical Associate, Department of Psychiatry, Perelman School of Medicine, University of Pennsylvania, Philadelphia, Pennsylvania

Alix Vann, PhD, Psychologist in private practice, Brisbane, Queensland, Australia

ACKNOWLEDGMENTS

We were encouraged by many psychotherapists, students, and colleagues to further our project of making psychodynamic therapy pragmatic and understandable by showing how the ideas we developed and expressed in our first book, *Psychodynamic Therapy: A Guide to Evidence-Based Practice* (2010), are put into practice. In response, we asked colleagues whose clinical work was influenced by those ideas if they would be willing to write up their work with patients.

This casebook took off one evening over a lasagna dinner at RFS's house in 2011, with seven or eight colleagues attending in person and several others joining by Skype from Colorado, Texas, and Australia. We discussed the project and there was unanimous support. The chapter authors were inspired by the idea of writing about the kinds of patients that everyone would recognize—regular people with problems, strengths, and vulnerabilities—not ideal patients with lots of resources. (They also thought the lasagna was not bad!) We decided that the authors would use a consistent format to describe their patients and the treatment, but that each therapist's and patient's voice would dictate the specifics of the write-up, and we hoped the uniqueness of each therapeutic encounter would shine through.

We were very pleased that The Guilford Press, and our always encouraging and discriminating editor, Jim Nageotte, wanted to publish the work. We thank them for their support and guidance, and for their commitment to new ideas about psychodynamic therapy. Jim reminded us of the importance of directness, clarity, and parsimony in narrating a case, and this has been enormously helpful.

We sincerely thank the authors of the chapters who selected treatment experiences that they found interesting and challenging. We did not ask them to present patients who did well or those who did not. Many of the authors are from the University of Pennsylvania, where RFS is on the faculty and JPB was for many years. Others had read our previous book and expressed interest in being part of the project.

We thank the patients who gave permission for their stories to be written about, and we are so grateful to them for letting their therapists into their lives and letting us all in as well. They have taught us so much and helped us all understand more about life, love, loss, suffering, and resilience.

The University of Pennsylvania psychiatry residents and psychology graduate students, Adelphi students and graduate students, and the many participants in workshops, Grand Rounds, and courses we have done all over the United States and in Europe and Australia have been an inspiration to us. In an era when psychodynamic therapy has lost ground in insurance reimbursement, educational settings, and popular culture to some degree, it has been a pleasure to know how many people are interested in learning about it and are committed to making it one of the essential therapeutic choices for patients in the future.

Justina Kaminskaite Dillon and Sigal Zilcha-Mano, students of JPB at Adelphi, helped us by reading chapters and providing valuable editorial and content feedback. They helped us develop an appreciation for what would be useful for both beginning and more advanced therapists to see in this book.

RFS would like to thank Tony Rostain and Dwight Evans in the University of Pennsylvania Department of Psychiatry. Other colleagues, residents, and staff, especially Michele Cepparulo and Cassie Sacco, make the department an enormously supportive and generative place to teach, learn, and practice. Alan Gruenberg, Margaret Ann Price, James Hetznecker, and Pace Duckett have offered, as always, their clinical wisdom, perspective, and collegiality.

JPB would like to thank Provost Gayle D. Insler and President Robert A. Scott at Adelphi University for supporting his scholarship and his colleague deans who teach him daily about new and different ways of handling his job.

Our wives, Ronnie and Smadar, are our greatest supporters and they have encouraged us in all of our endeavors. We are so grateful to them. We thank our children (and, for JPB, two grandchildren) for their love and support and for helping us be our best.

CONTENTS

INTRODUCTION

RICHARD F. SUMMERS
JACQUES P. BARBER

Psychotherapy is a personal exchange between two people that has a beginning, middle, and end. The patient and therapist come together and form a connection that spins out an arc of emotion, experience and memory that neither could quite anticipate, and then they wind down and separate, hopefully with the patient feeling better and the therapist wiser.

This book is a collection of descriptions of psychotherapy written by psychotherapists who have been influenced by the conceptualization of psychodynamic therapy described in our first book, *Psychodynamic Therapy: A Guide to Evidence-Based Practice* (Summers & Barber, 2010). We present the reality of psychotherapy and focus on what is essential in driving a patient and therapist forward toward an active, energizing, and healthy interaction that results in change.

The raison d'être of this book is to counter the accumulated layers of sclerotic theory and outdated technique that weigh down the development of psychodynamic theory and praxis, and to contribute to the evolution of clinical conceptualizations and practices that are clear, succinct, structured, and based, as much as possible, on evidence. Our goals are to exemplify the model we previously articulated through detailed case histories, facilitate learning of our method, provide a tool for teaching and supervision, and help trainees get exposure to more cases.

The variety of therapy experiences illustrated here will help to explain the basic principles of the psychodynamic model, show their utility, and reveal some limitations. We start this volume with two chapters summarizing our conceptualization of contemporary psychodynamic theory and technique and follow with twelve case descriptions.

The emphasis on cases in this book comes from our experience in teaching about psychodynamic therapy and shows our commitment to using case histories as a learning tool. It takes quite a while for trainees to treat enough patients to really understand the psychodynamic model and its application, and to see the arc of treatment enough times to understand how to set it in motion. Teaching and training must explain the theory early and effectively, but it must also convey an intuitive, visceral grasp of how a treatment begins, does its magic, and ends.

Improving the pedagogy for any psychotherapy, but particularly for psychodynamic therapy, is especially timely for several reasons:

1. The evidence base for psychodynamic therapy has increasing heft (Barber, Muran, McCarthy, & Keefe, 2013), even though the field struggles against the powerful headwinds of research funding bias and medical economics.
2. The current generation of mental health professionals is frequently not adequately exposed to and trained in pragmatic psychodynamic therapy techniques.
3. There is some cause for optimism about clinical opportunities for psychodynamic therapists in the future and for the reversal of the powerful trend away from this treatment.

PERSONAL REFLECTIONS

We were struck by many readers' reactions to *Psychodynamic Therapy: A Guide to Evidence-Based Practice*. They told us the book spoke to how they were trying to practice, and they recognized their worldview and sensibility in it—pragmatic and engaged, concerned with the scientific evidence base yet passionate about the importance of letting people tell and rework their stories, committed to patient empowerment and transparency, and relying on an active stance by the therapist.

Many trainees and early career therapists said the book influenced their thinking and identity as therapists, and this sparked their interest in exploring psychodynamic ideas and contributing to their evolution. We were, of course, excited by these developments and wanted to take the next step. We wanted to illustrate and refine the model. We asked younger colleagues and former trainees to present cases that would reflect our psychodynamic model and that would serve as the scaffold for the fleshing out of these ideas. We selected cases that are typical of the problems and responses that therapists meet in real clinical settings.

Another experience contributed to the inspiration for this casebook. As a therapist in a randomized clinical trial comparing the efficacy of psychodynamic therapy versus cognitive-behavioral therapy versus applied relaxation therapy for panic disorder, one of us (RFS) had access to video recordings of a number of time-limited, complete psychotherapies with permission from the patients to use these records for teaching. One of the treatments (24 hours of recorded psychotherapy) was edited down to 90 minutes, comprising a series of 6- to 10-minute segments culled to illustrate the development, sweep, and resolution of the therapeutic encounter. Psychotherapy involves periods of quiescence and wandering reflection punctuated by moments of intense awareness, engagement and salience, and the resulting edited film certainly focused on these exciting moments, a bit like the TV series *In Treatment*.

This video was used to teach psychiatry residents and other trainees at the University of Pennsylvania and around the world. Students and clinicians watching the film reflected on the aerial view of the arc of the psychotherapy provided by the edited sequence, and appreciated the sped-up experience of learning about what happens over the entire course of treatment. Gaining this experience usually requires a much greater expenditure of time. We hope exposure to these case histories will provide the same type of "big-picture" educational experience for our readers that viewing the edited psychotherapy did for our trainees.

Many psychiatrist and psychologist colleagues with diverse practices came forward with an interest in contributing case histories. We regard each of the contributors to this collection as talented and skillful, and are pleased to be able to illustrate their work. They have taken a risk, as all authors do, in displaying their work, and taken additional risk in providing their self-reflections and assessments of the treatments. We believe honest self-reflection and sharing help to refine and develop one's craft. Our chapter authors, we believe, give an important gift in sharing their personal observations.

The cases presented in this book come from a variety of settings (e.g., training clinics, private practice) and include patients with a range of function. Because our model relies heavily on the notion of the core psychodynamic problem and the critical importance of identifying the problem early in treatment as a basis for active collaboration between patient and therapist, we include cases that illustrate all six of the core problems we have described—depression, obsessionality, fear of abandonment, low self-esteem, panic anxiety, and trauma. While change strategies and transference–countertransference enactments are fully discussed in the cases, it is really the recognition of the core problem and the striking of a therapeutic alliance around work on that problem that moves the therapy from the beginning to the end and takes its place as a fundamental anchor of our model.

Some of the cases are much more specifically connected to the model, while others are consistent with it but have other important theoretical and practical influences. The cases are naturalistic in the sense that they reflect clinical work designed and implemented by a mental health professional in settings where the patient has considerable freedom to choose the goals, type, and technique of therapy.

A NEW WAY OF LEARNING ABOUT PSYCHODYNAMIC THERAPY

Learning psychotherapy has been likened to other kinds of complex skill acquisition. The Dreyfus brothers' model, which has broad acceptance in business as well as medical education settings (Dreyfus & Dreyfus, 1980), identifies consecutive stages of skill acquisition, including novice, competent, and expert levels. These levels reflect sequential accumulation of skills, knowledge, and their application. Thus, learning psychotherapy entails many steps and hours of training to develop the necessary expertise to treat patients.

We suggest that psychodynamic therapy education and training have traditionally been robust and effective for those therapists who are already interested and have a reasonable knowledge base. But the early phases of learning, including initial exposure, early practice of technique, and the development of an initial synthesis and style, have been left to nature. The techniques for teaching novice skills and facilitating movement toward competence have not been as fully developed and attended to as the methods for further development of experienced psychodynamic therapists. This is a gap we want to bridge with this book.

Indeed, we believe that learning about psychodynamic therapy requires three elements: (1) *framework*—a clear and concise model; (2) *feeling*—an experiential immersion in what happens in therapy, including a big-picture appreciation of the arc of treatment; and (3) *freedom*— the opportunity to practice in a safe, nonjudgmental setting with lots of feedback and the opportunity to explore, experience, make mistakes, and reflect. We see this casebook as a contribution to the "feeling" part of the learning experience—it will allow you, the reader, to dive into twelve psychotherapeutic encounters. You will be exposed to the struggles of twelve patients, the formulation of their core psychodynamic problems, and the techniques for translating all of that information and experience into a focused treatment that leads to change and, ultimately, the end of therapy. The summary of our pragmatic psychodynamic model in Chapters 1 and 2 will prepare you for that.

The process of identifying with mentors and supervisors, and combining and transforming the lessons from their behavior and approach into one's own unique synthesis, is a lifelong process. In tough clinical situations, many of us find ourselves reflecting on what our analysts, our therapists, or particular favorite supervisors and valued colleagues would have said if they had had to deal with what we are now facing. Or what we imagine they would have said! Reading the cases here provides an opportunity to add to that process. You will consider the sensibility, tone, decisions, and strategies of each therapist and can incorporate those features that resonate with you into your own work.

Written cases have advantages over videotaped sessions. They protect privacy much better, and are a more processed mode of presentation than video. The author can highlight the essential themes and experiences and create a picture that emphasizes the figure in relation to the background, just like an artist's rendering brings out realities a photograph cannot. Despite these obvious advantages, we are all aware that a written case is clearly a production of the therapist and reflects to some degree his or her needs, biases, strengths, and limitations. We introduce each case with a few paragraphs of observations in italics about some important aspects of the treatment and make relevant connections with our model.

Maintaining confidentiality is essential to therapy. Most cases presented in this book are confidential in that all of the identifiable personal information has been changed to protect the privacy of the patients. Some cases are fictionalized by combining the stories of several real patients so that the material makes psychological and psychotherapeutic sense but does not actually reflect the history of a particular person. Most stick close to the real experience with the patient although important details are changed and disguised to protect privacy, and informed consent was provided.

HOW TO READ THE CASES

Each case is written in a relatively standard format, with a chief complaint and presenting problem, history, psychodynamic formulation, course of treatment, termination, and assessment of progress. But that's where the similarities end!

We each found that an essential part of our own learning as psychotherapists took place while reading. One reads about a patient's history and life experiences, arrayed over a timeline, notices patterns repeating and changing, and sees a therapist straining to understand, characterize, communicate, and facilitate. Reading other people's cases is a rich opportunity to self-reflect and understand more fully one's own clinical experiences. This may involve remembering complicated and confusing experiences with patients and seeing them in a new light with a deeper awareness of one's own feelings or an increased empathic understanding of the patient.

We hope you will be able to tap into this self-reflective reading and learning experience and see it for the refreshing, invigorating, although sometimes anxious, experience that it is. Let your mind wander, notice the moments in the stories you return to and the things you struggle with, and consider your own identity and style as a therapist.

On a less ethereal level, we encourage you to ask a number of questions of each case to help you read actively. You may want to stop for a minute or two in the midst of a chapter to consider them to help keep your reading fresh and open.

- What is the essential story? What are the key aspects of the patient's history and why did the patient seek treatment? What happened over the course of therapy and what kind of change occurred in the patient and in the relationship with the therapist?

- What did it feel like to be the patient? What was his or her everyday experience, the particular type of suffering and discontent? When was the patient particularly vulnerable and compromised and what were his or her strengths? How well did you feel like you could understand the patient's subjective experience? Did you feel the therapist was able to?

- What was it like to be the therapist? What was interesting and exciting, and what was anxiety-producing, frustrating, or confusing? Can you imagine yourself in the therapist's shoes?

- What did you think of the therapist's conceptualization of the core psychodynamic problem? How different were the patient's and therapist's understanding and did these views converge as the treatment went on?

- How did the therapeutic alliance develop? Can you identify the components of the alliance—goal, task, and bond? What do you learn from the therapist's decisions about handling the obstacles to the alliance? Can you see the difference between the therapeutic alliance and the positive feeling shared by the patient and therapist? Can you distinguish between the therapeutic alliance and the transference and countertransference reactions?

• How did the patient change? Do you think there was a substantial change or an incremental one? Was it a change in how the patient feels, sees the world, or behaves? Was the amount of change reasonable for this patient? Did you expect more or less?

• Was the treatment, and the arc of the interaction between therapist and patient, predictable? As you read, are you forming hypotheses about what will happen next, and are your hypotheses accurate? Does the core problem formulation help in your predictions?

• How did reading the case stimulate your own introspection, either about being a therapist or a patient? Did the case authors' self-observations help you be more self-aware and honest in your own reflections?

• Did the therapist adhere closely to the model we have proposed, and was there a clear application of these ideas and techniques? Are there other important influences on the therapist that are apparent and how did that change the treatment?

It is our hope that these questions, which we should ask of ourselves every day in our clinical work, will help keep you in an active and critical (in the constructive sense of the word!) stance as you read. You might try looking at the questions again after you read each chapter and use them as a study guide.

REFERENCES

Barber, J. P., Muran, J. C., McCarthy, K. S., & Keefe, R. J. (2013). Research on psychodynamic therapies. In M. J. Lambert (Ed.). *Bergin and Garfield's handbook of psychotherapy and behavior change* (6th ed., pp. 443–494). New York: Wiley.

Dreyfus, S. E., & Dreyfus, H. L. (1980, February). *A five-stage model of the mental activities involved in directed skill acquisition.* Washington, DC: Storming Media.

Summers, R. F., & Barber, J. P. (2010). *Psychodynamic therapy: A guide to evidence-based practice.* New York: Guilford Press.

CHAPTER 1

PRAGMATIC PSYCHODYNAMIC PSYCHOTHERAPY

The Therapeutic Alliance and the Core Psychodynamic Problem

RICHARD F. SUMMERS
JACQUES P. BARBER

Our model of psychodynamic therapy, which we have referred to as pragmatic psychodynamic psychotherapy (PPP), is based on a the traditional conflict model of mental life and highlights the therapeutic alliance, core psychodynamic problem and formulation, as well as patient education and transparency, integration with other synergistic treatment modalities, and an active, engaged stance for the therapist (Summers & Barber, 2010). It differs from traditional psychodynamic psychotherapy, which is less focused, more hierarchical, diagnostically nonspecific, and not as easily integrated (conceptually and technically) with psychopharmacology and other concurrent treatments. PPP is an umbrella notion that comprises an overarching model and technique that can be found in general clinical practice as well as in specific evidence-based psychodynamic treatments like Luborsky's supportive–expressive therapy (Luborsky, 1984) and panic–focused psychodynamic therapy (Busch, Milrod, Singer, & Aronson, 2011; Milrod, Busch, Cooper, & Shapiro, 1997).

The history of psychotherapy over the past century helps to place this model in a broader context. Over the last several decades, there has been greater interest in specific techniques and a movement away from more generalized models, that is, from "one size fits all" to therapies tailored to particular diagnoses and symptoms. There is more attention to how treatments are tailored to diagnoses and individual patients, and a refreshing interest in the patient's experience of the therapeutic relationship and treatment setting. When we look back at the history of psychotherapy in the late 20th and early 21st century, the intense focus on scientific understanding of psychotherapy outcomes and processes will probably stand out as the most salient new development in psychotherapy, including in psychodynamic therapy (e.g., Barber, Muran, McCarthy, & Keefe, 2013).

Our model of psychodynamic therapy attempts to make a series of connections between the burgeoning database from treatment outcomes studies (about psychotherapy in general, and psychodynamic therapy in particular) and the theory and application of psychodynamic ideas. Thus, PPP was developed to distill out and identify the essential features of effective psychodynamic therapy, and then to assess the degree of evidence supporting these building blocks of the therapeutic model. A detailed discussion of the components of psychodynamic therapy in our model is beyond the scope of this casebook and is found in Summers and Barber (2010).

In this chapter and the next, we will focus on five of the essential building blocks of the model: the therapeutic alliance, the core psychodynamic problem, the psychodynamic formulation, strategies for facilitating change, and termination. This will provide the context for reading the cases.

THE THERAPEUTIC ALLIANCE

The first of the five components of psychodynamic therapy we will review is the therapeutic alliance. The notion of the therapeutic alliance captures the emerging collaborative enterprise that joins the patient and therapist in their work. It is the here-and-now working relationship that is designed to neutralize painful, outdated neurotic experiences with current strengths, and the fulcrum upon which rests the opportunity for change. It is referred to variously as the therapeutic, working, or helping alliance, and has been the subject of much empirical research (e.g., Barber, Muran, McCarthy, & Keefe, 2013; Muran & Barber, 2010).

Freud (1912) foreshadowed the now widely accepted idea that the therapeutic relationship is important for the success of the therapy by commenting on the positive feelings that develop between doctor and patient. Later psychoanalysts such as Greenson (1967) and Zetzel

(1956) distinguished between the "real" and adaptive dimensions of the treatment relationship and its transferential and fantasy-laden aspects. Although the alliance concept emerged in the psychoanalytic literature, the importance of the collaborative relationship between patient and therapist is regarded as crucial by therapists from many theoretical backgrounds.

Goal, Task, and Bond

Edward Bordin (1979) identified three components of the therapeutic alliance and sought to operationalize these notions and apply them across the psychotherapies. He understood the therapeutic alliance as a mutual construction of the patient and therapist with three elements: shared *goals*, an understanding of the *tasks* each person must perform in the relationship, and an attachment *bond*. He observed that different psychotherapies call upon different aspects of the therapeutic alliance at different points over the course of treatment.

Goal refers to the alignment of purpose between the therapist and patient. What is the patient working toward, what does he or she want to understand or change? What aspect of life is he or she concerned about, and what does he or she want to do about it? The therapist must appreciate the patient's goals and accept them, or work with the patient to change them. For example, if the therapist sees the problem as depression and sensitivity to rejection and loss, but the patient thinks the problem is a parenting issue with a difficult child and an unhelpful husband, not only are the pictures of the problem different, but the goals will also reflect that difference. The therapist may address the depression, expecting the life problems to improve as a result, but the patient will feel confused by the therapist's interest in her past and other relationships, and probably criticized, too.

Task refers to the jobs each member of the therapeutic dyad must perform. The patient's task is to come to the sessions, express thoughts and feelings honestly and openly, observe them, and try to listen to and accept the therapist's observations. There is also the ineffable task of taking responsibility for one's self and trying to change. The therapist's job, on the other hand, is to work hard to listen and understand, focus and attend, put aside personal biases and assumptions as much as possible, conceptualize the patient's problems and effectively share this understanding (Luborsky, 1984). The therapist should also facilitate new perceptions of self and of others and new behavioral responses to the same old troubling situations. The therapist must let the patient guide the treatment, but provide guidance, help, and knowledge.

Bond refers to the emotional link between patient and therapist. Does the patient feel connected to the therapist and therapy, and is there a sense of warmth and empathy? From the therapist's perspective, is there emotional engagement and the mix of caring with objectivity and separateness that allows us to do our best work?

Across many studies, the alliance correlates with psychodynamic treatment outcome (r = .275, Barber et al., 2013). In the field of psychotherapy research, it is difficult to isolate important process variables with a high degree of confidence, and the alliance stands out as a clearly valid construct although it accounts quantitatively for a small amount of the variance in outcome.

Transference

The psychoanalytic tradition usefully distinguished between the therapeutic alliance and the *transference*. The alliance is the here and now collaborative development of two people working together in the present, while the transference is the array of feelings, thoughts, perceptions, and fantasies the patient has about the therapist based on earlier life experiences, especially with primary caretakers during childhood. The former is a product of the patient's adult and mature mind, while the latter is a result of earlier important relationships, old grooved-in patterns of relating, and the weight of personal emotional history. Understanding the transference is a gold mine in psychodynamic therapy, because it allows the patient and therapist to see and experience old reactions in an immediate real way in the office. However, observing and identifying the transference in the office is often confusing for beginning therapists as it may be difficult to distinguish between the patient's feelings and perceptions about the therapist based on the constructed therapeutic alliance and the feelings that have roots in the transference. For example, is a patient who feels criticized and judged by the therapist, feeling there is no room to express her thoughts without criticism, showing a problem with the therapeutic alliance because of misaligned goals and a misunderstanding about tasks? Or is this a transferential reaction based on the patient's fantasy that opening up to someone else and feeling dependent inevitably results in being judged and demeaned? That will be for you and the patient to figure out! You will see in the cases here the intertwining of these elements and the therapists' decisions about when to try to address problems in the alliance and when to discuss and interpret the transference. These are important moments in psychotherapy, and dealing with potential and actual ruptures in the therapeutic alliance is a key skill that can be learned through understanding and practice.

Ruptures

Empathy, attunement, education, early recognition of the patient's core problem, along with a caring, engaged professional demeanor, help the therapist to build the alliance. But, potential ruptures in the alliance (Safran, Muran, & Eubacks-Carter, 2011) are inevitable because no therapist is perfect, and the transference always interferes. Whether it is excessive respect and the need to please, or disappointment and feelings of rejection, the patient's perception of the therapist must include transferential distortions that are not current, logical, or rational, and are at odds with the present reality. The therapist will inevitably trip the wire of the patient's negative transference and provoke some type of anger, frustration, disappointment, or loss. Ruptures are practically inevitable (Safran et al., 2011) because those feelings are lying dormant (or not so dormant) in the patient and the intensity and intimacy of the therapeutic situation results in their coming closer to the surface.

We see understanding the therapeutic alliance, and its relationship to transference, as crucial, and we support a variety of approaches to improve training in this area (Summers & Barber, 2003), including greater educational attention to alliance building and rupture repair and the use of therapeutic alliance rating scales to help trainees learn more about their patients' perceptions of them.

THE CORE PSYCHODYNAMIC PROBLEM

The second building block of PPP is diagnosing the core psychodynamic problem (Summers & Barber, 2010). We contend that six core psychodynamic problems (Table 1.1)—depression, obsessionality, fear of abandonment, low self-esteem, panic anxiety, and trauma—account for roughly 80–90% of those who are appropriately treated with psychodynamic psychotherapy. We see these as the essential narratives for understanding most of the problems patients bring to us. There are surely other ways of categorizing problems (general schemes and psychodynamic schemes), but these six have the virtue of seeming to "carve nature at its joints," that is, stay close to the phenomena patients describe, and allow us to connect psychodynamic conceptualizations with descriptive diagnoses like those in DSM-5.

These six psychodynamic problems have either empirical outcome data (depression, panic anxiety, fear of abandonment) or clinical experience to support their inclusion on our list, and represent the key conditions that can be well treated by psychodynamic therapy. Certainly they are not the only problems that respond to dynamic treatment, but they

TABLE 1.1. Core Psychodynamic Problems

- Depression
- Obsessionality
- Fear of abandonment
- Low self-esteem
- Panic anxiety
- Trauma

Note. From Summers and Barber (2010). Copyright 2010 by The Guilford Press. Reprinted by permission.

are the most common ones. While we suggest that psychodynamic therapy is effective for these conditions, we certainly recognize that other treatments, such as cognitive-behavioral therapy or medication, may be as effective.

The process of recognizing these problems in the clinic may be difficult at times. Some patients easily fit the profile of one problem well, and some have features of more than one. The case histories to come will illustrate the value and some of the challenges of using the core psychodynamic problem to understand a patient and organize the treatment.

We use the term *core psychodynamic problem* to denote problems with common underlying patterns. The traditional psychoanalytic diagnoses—for example, obsessional neurosis, hysterical character, and phobic neurosis among others—had characteristic symptoms, identifiable (although inferred) dynamics, and hypothesized etiologies (Fenichel, 1945). These entities were regarded as specific forms of pathology. But, the classic psychoanalytic diagnostic system was unreliable and difficult to apply clinically because of its reliance on a high degree of inference. In addition, the therapy was not tailored to the diagnosis. One man's obsession was another man's phobia, and the distinction was not very important because they both required the same treatment technique (Greenson, 1967).

We take a heuristic approach to diagnosis, aiming for what is clinically useful. The core problems are explanations that will help patients feel better. This is different from the traditional psychoanalytic nosology and from the DSM tradition that tries to divide psychopathology into many different specific disorders. Instead, we describe explanations that cut across different forms of depression, for example. In this sense, our framework is closer to the increasingly popular transdiagnostic approach recently recommended by Barlow (2011) and others.

Most associated DSM-5 diagnoses	Psychodynamic treatment goals	Character strengths affected	Therapeutic alliance issues
Major depression, persistent depressive disorder	Decreased vulnerability to abandonment, decreased self-punishment	Courage, humanity, transcendence	Empathy, encouragement, instillation of hope, education about depression
Obsessive–compulsive personality disorder, subclinical obsessive–compulsive disorder	Decreased guilt, increased tolerance of affective experience	Wisdom and knowledge, humanity, transcendence	Psychoeducation about therapy and importance of affects, elicitation of feelings
Atypical depression, Cluster B personality disorder, somatization disorder, some eating disorders	More stable image of self and other, decreased mood reactivity, increased stability of relationships	Justice, temperance	Empathy, development of contractual relationship leading to relationship development
Narcissistic personality disorder, persistent depressive disorder	More accurate and positive self-image, increased ability to tolerate vulnerability	Wisdom and knowledge, humanity, temperance	Attention to empathic bond
Panic disorder with or without agoraphobia	Increased independence and ability to be assertive without overwhelming anxiety and anger	Courage, transcendence	More frequent sessions, empathic attention to episodes of panic, close exploration of precipitants, psychoeducation about panic, ability to tolerate necessary discomfort
Posttraumatic stress disorder, Cluster B personality disorder, atypical depression, somatization disorder, some eating disorders	Increased sense of security and empowerment, increased healthy trust in relationships	Courage, humanity	Clearly spelled-out boundaries and expectations, mutual respect, attention to fact and reality

(continued)

TABLE 1.2. (*continued*)

Depression	Obsessionality	Abandonment fear	Low self-esteem	Panic anxiety	Trauma
		Typical resistances			
Overwhelming affects, hopelessness, passivity	Characteristic obsessional defenses (intellectualization, isolation of affect, reaction formation, etc.), overvaluing of thought over feeling	Fear of abandonment, premature ending of therapy	Inevitable ruptures in empathy	Dependency, avoidance	Fear leading to reenactment of traumatic situation
		Technique issues			
Initial phase of empathy, support, encouragement of function; second phase of identification of key themes of abandonment/loss, and conflict over resentment about losses; maintenance phase related to early recognition of increased conflict and planning for effective solutions	Active listening, focus on feelings, gentle but firm confrontation, attention to anger and guilt, some directiveness, use of patient's cognitive skills to help identify patterns	Concept of containment, appropriate management strategies, mixing of supportive and exploratory interventions; progression from relationship development to working through dependency to true working alliance	Consistent emphasis on ruptures in empathy, repair and recognition of this continuing vulnerability	Identification of precipitants, challenging of avoidance; interpretation of conflict associated with panic, focusing primarily on precipitants but connecting to historical antecedents and transference; encouragement of widened scope of behavior; tolerate resurgence of separation reaction at termination	Collaborative, flexible attitude, focus on empowerment and realistic perceptions, truth-telling, respect for boundaries

18

Typical transferences

Abandonment, dependency, idealization, anger	Controlling, passive-aggressive, "resistant," anger and hostility, anxiety about being controlled, struggle for freedom and autonomy	Abandonment, rage, dependency, projective identification, micro-psychotic episodes especially related to transference abandonment	Mirroring, idealizing, twinship	Separation, loss, abandonment; anger about loss; fear of further loss or retribution because of anger	Lack of trust, fear and vigilance, rage at lack of help, need to control therapist, reenactment of trauma

Typical countertransferences

Rescue fantasies, feeling incompetent, sucked dry	Frustration, feeling of being controlled, retaliatory fantasies, boredom, distance, futility	Helplessness, anger, guilt, impulse toward boundary crossing	Rescue fantasy, grandiosity, anger at feeling defeated, boredom	Maternal, rescue and caretaking; frustration with dependency and rejection	Identification with victim, helplessness, identification with perpetrator, bystander/witness guilt, secondary posttraumatic stress disorder, confusion

Note. Adapted from Summers and Barber (2010). Copyright 2010 by The Guilford Press. Adapted by permission.

problems prepares you for reading the cases which include patients with all six problems. You will quickly see that the problems include overlapping characteristics, like a Venn diagram, as there are only so many sources of emotional pain. This overlap is reasonable because we are not developing a diagnostic scheme of illnesses, but rather a set of heuristics that allow the patient to develop a coherent story that will facilitate his or her ability to change. We have followed the same order of presentation for the description of the core problems in this chapter as we have for the cases that illustrate the problems in the rest of the book.

In our review of the core problems, we focus on the symptoms, psychodynamic conceptualization, issues in the development of the alliance, therapeutic goals, techniques, and transference–countertransference reactions associated with each problem. Of course, you will need to learn quite a bit more about each problem to be able to fully conduct the treatment, but each capsule summary will provide a roadmap for the path to be traveled.

Depression: Loss and Guilt

Depression is one of the most common problems that bring people to therapy (World Health Organization, 2008). It is a broadly defined condition that includes a mixture of sadness, loss, melancholy, boredom, frustration, irritability, fear, abandonment, and hopelessness. For the core problem of depression, the pervasive affective experience of sadness and loss is central. Although feelings of sadness, low mood, or loss are ubiquitous and almost everyone experiences them from time to time, their persistence can start a vicious cycle of negativity—sadness, loss, withdrawal, demoralization, and increased self-criticism—which leads to further withdrawal and negative outlook. The neurovegetative symptoms of depression, including changes in sleep, appetite, and energy, along with problems in focus and concentration and the loss of ability to enjoy oneself, suicidal thinking, and loss of sexual interest, may co-exist with prominent subjective feelings of worthlessness, pessimism, and sadness.

Busch et al.'s (2004) cogent formulation provides a useful psychodynamic conceptualization for depression. Their synthesis suggests that early losses lead to frustration and anger, which inevitably result in guilt about the angry feelings and wishes. This guilt makes a person feel badly about him- or herself. Restitutive efforts to manage the low self-esteem lead to neediness and unrealistic expectations from others. These expectations inevitably turn out badly as the disappointments that follow inflated expectations lead to feeling rejected and unlovable, and this in turn reinforces the guilt and low self-esteem.

This historic pattern is restimulated by subsequent losses and adverse experience.

The therapeutic alliance with patients presenting with depression develops rapidly because the patient is scared and suffering. Feelings of dependency, especially when the therapist is supplying energy, hope, and constructive attention, will certainly make for a rapid and strong attachment. But, as we have seen, developing a good alliance requires more than positive emotion for the therapist. It means the patient must perform the necessary tasks of self-reflection and trying new things, and the therapist must take a practical perspective and push the patient to be as active as possible, both in the hard work of therapy and in the engagement with the world. These tasks are a formidable challenge for a depressed, negative, and self-critical patient, and the therapist needs to be patient, educating him or her about the process, and helpful in supporting the patient in taking on the responsibility of being in therapy. The therapeutic goal is to help the depressed patient feel less self-critical and less vulnerable to loss.

Technique

The first phase of treatment involves building of the therapeutic alliance as well as behavioral mobilization and activation. In treating depression, more than the other six core problems, there is a need to support and educate the patient, and encourage his or her increased activity in a pragmatic and sensitive way. Just as internal change can cause behavioral change, changes in behavior may result in an altered experience of self and other. (We discuss this bidirectional effect at greater length below in the section on change.)

Educating the patient about depression is rather straightforward. You may explain that upsetting feelings, especially about loss, have taken on a life of their own, and lead the patient to become preoccupied with negative, hopeless thoughts, and neurovegetative symptoms. Patients often find it helpful to learn there is usually a mix of genetic vulnerability and life stressors that precipitate and maintain the depression, and especially that the prognosis is quite good with a variety of treatments, including psychodynamic therapy.

The second, and more specifically psychodynamic, phase of therapy focuses on identifying the key themes of abandonment and loss, resentment about the loss and subsequent conflict over this resentment. Patient and therapist work together to help the patient recall and reexperience important earlier losses, explore the feelings of loss, guilt, anger, and self-criticism and see the dynamics as they may have actually played out in the patient's life. Busch et al. (2004) provide the model for connecting the loss, anger, guilt, and attempt to restore self-esteem through relationships that are disappointing because of excessive expectations.

The third phase of the psychodynamic therapy of depression, once the symptoms have substantially abated, focuses on consolidating the understanding achieved in the second phase, and on identifying and observing the depressive pattern of loss, guilt, disappointment, and low self-esteem. New and more realistic perceptions are considered and refined, and the patient is supported in finding different and healthier behavioral responses to these increasingly realistic responses to relationships and activities. There is also attention to early recognition of conflict-stimulating situations, skills in managing such situations, and increasing understanding of the differences between old perceptions and feelings and current adult awareness.

Transference and Countertransference

The most frequent transference reaction of depressed patients is abandonment and hunger for a closer connection with the therapist. This transference pattern is especially common for patients with great feelings of emptiness and loss. It is frequently associated with a dependency reaction, where the patient feels profoundly helpless and has a desperate sense of needing the therapist. Some depressed patients idealize their therapists, and see them as endless sources of emotional supplies. But, the other side of the dependent transference reaction is anger and disappointment. Here the patient is filled with a sense of rejection and disappointment, and previous losses are reexperienced with the therapist now in the role of the absent or hurtful parent. Patients with substantial anger and guilt are more likely to experience the therapist as critical and rejecting.

There are many kinds of countertransference responses a therapist may have, but there are some that are typical with patients with particular core problems. It is common to develop a rescue fantasy in response to working with depressed patients. This fantasy reflects a powerful personal belief that one can make the patient better. This countertransference reaction may involve the therapist feeling he or she can help the patient become whole through their close relationship, and the feeling that the therapist's interest and warmth will make the patient feel life is worth living. Some patients feel so deprived on entering therapy, and are so pleased with the therapist's attention, that they unconsciously reinforce the therapist's caretaking behavior by making him or her feel like a savior. Of course, this can go too far. There is a big difference between trying to help by exercising professional and personal skills, and being driven by a feeling that you have the special mission to rescue a desperate patient. After all, every patient must take responsibility and do work on his or her own, and the therapist's job is to support that. Other counter-transference reactions include feeling angry at the level of demand of the patient, or feeling exhausted and depleted by not being able to nurture the patient back to health.

Obsessionality: Controlling Feelings

Obsessional patients are preoccupied with rules, ideas, and procedures, and are typically distant from their feelings. It is not that they do not have feelings—they do have very strong emotions, but they regard emotions as "inconvenient" and upsetting. Obsessionals aspire to focus only on what is logical and rational, and what adheres to rules.

The main explanatory concept in the psychoanalytic literature on obsessionality is struggle and discomfort with aggressive feelings and the use of specific defenses to manage them. Originally, psychoanalytic writers proposed that obsessionality had its origins in problems occurring during the anal phase of development (Freud, 1908) and pointed to the obsessional neurotics' tendency to value order, ritual, and thought over emotion, similar to the child's preoccupation with these qualities during toilet training. Subsequent thinking emphasized the obsessional patient's notion that anger is bad and must be gotten rid of, controlled, and disarmed (A. Freud, 1966).

Anger is often associated with guilt, and this seems especially true for these patients, who try to manage their anger and guilt through the alchemy of obsessional defenses. The five obsessional defenses are (1) *intellectualization*, the focus on complex cognitive processes rather than gut feelings; (2) *isolation of affect*, the separation of thoughts from feelings; (3) *reaction formation*, the substitution of a positive feeling for a negative one; (4) *displacement*, the shifting of feelings and conflicts from one situation onto another that is unrelated (e.g., road rage after a family argument); and (5) *doing and undoing*, the tendency to express something (verbally or through behavior) and then undo it by expressing the opposite. Each of these defenses operates unconsciously and results in the patient feeling less angry, guilty, and conflicted.

Salzman (1968) observed that patients with obsessional problems maintain, and feel a need to maintain, strict control over their emotions. They also control others in order to control their experience of relationships.

In summary, all of the psychodynamic conceptualizations of obsessionality include the notion that the patient struggles with anger, feels guilty, and tries to control his or her inner experience as well as the world around them. So, it is not a surprise that the biggest dilemma in developing a therapeutic alliance with obsessional patients is their difficulty in tolerating and experiencing emotions. Anger is the most difficult emotion, and obsessional people worry they will lose control and their anger will come spilling out with disastrous results. They tend to feel this has already happened, which leads them to worry about retaliation by others. The goal of psychodynamic therapy for obsessional patients is to experience more pleasure, spontaneity, emotion, and autonomy, and less sense of pressure, guilt, anger, and fear.

Technique

All psychotherapy patients may benefit from psychoeducation, an explanation of the treatment and how it will help with the problem. Obsessional patients are particularly interested in this preparation for therapy because of their love of rules, procedures, and ideas. A good, simple explanation of what psychotherapy is, how it is done, and how change occurs will set the stage for treatment. The patient's main responsibility—talking about thoughts and feelings as they are happening—is emphasized as a simple prescription.

You must listen closely for emotional reactions and gently work to elicit them with obsessional patients by directly inquiring, tactfully pointing out their body language, and trying to open up the subjective experience of each type of feeling and each experience. In other words, the therapist needs to help the patient recognize the feeling that is being avoided. For example, "When X did not return your call, how did you feel?" or "When he asked you to take on that task, what was your reaction?" You may comment on typical reactions people have to situations the patient is in and ask him or her whether this resonates and helps him or her identify current feelings.

As the treatment continues, you can focus more on the feelings of resentment and anger, and ask what it feels like; for example, "What are you afraid of when you are feeling this way?" Emotional experiences are clarified and named. Active acceptance and explicit validation of the patient's feelings is helpful, as obsessional patients are harshly self-critical and prone to shame. It is important to remember that these patients are focused on what they *should* feel and do what they can to avoid what they *do* feel.

Treating obsessionality requires persistence and activity. Patients may debate a course of action over weeks, and it is important to encourage taking a chance and making a best guess. Later the impact of the decision can be examined and dissected. The obsessional patient's tendency to ruminate rather than act needs to be met with a firm guiding hand, encouraging practice and exploration of life, trying new behaviors, and experimenting. You can easily get into a control battle with these patients although you started with good therapeutic intentions. Therapists should do their best to guide and encourage with a light touch, avoiding a potential counterproductive control struggle. The goal of these techniques is to bring out the emerging conflicted emotions and support the patient's ability to tolerate them.

Transference and Countertransference

Obsessional patients need to control the therapy and the therapist because this allows them to control themselves and their feelings. They are trying to manage the possible emergence of bad and dangerous feelings. This need for control may account for the sometimes dry and detached feeling of the interaction. Obsessionals are highly sensitive to feeling controlled and may struggle for control to preserve their freedom and autonomy. They will rebel or avoid you as though you were set on stamping out their autonomy. They may test you or try to control you. There may be indirect expressions of anger and hostility, or it may be more obvious.

Feeling frustration with the patient and a sense that he or she is deflecting and not engaging with you is quite common. The therapist can feel angry and have the urge to push through the patient's carefully constructed defenses, being just as aggressive as the patient imagines he or she is. Or one may feel boredom and distance. Sometimes the therapeutic game of cat and mouse feels futile and pointless. One may find oneself responding to the patient's underlying anger, which is expressed indirectly or passive-aggressively, with more anger oneself.

Fear of Abandonment

Fear of abandonment involves insecure attachment to others with a painful vulnerability to separation. Patients with fear of abandonment are desperate to avoid feeling loss and aloneness. They try to tolerate these painful feelings but often revert to dysfunctional strategies to stay connected with others. If you constantly feel alone and are scared of losing what little you have, you may appear unstable to others because of the strategies you employ to stay secure. Some patients have quite chaotic behavior, but fear of abandonment also shows itself in functional individuals who have anxious inner experiences but manage to maintain relatively adaptive behavior.

The traditional psychodynamic and psychoanalytic literature draws a direct link between abandonment fears and the diagnosis of borderline personality disorder. There were originally two major psychodynamic frameworks used to understand fear of abandonment—Bowlby's

(1999/1982) attachment theory and Kernberg's object relations perspective (e.g., Kernberg, Selzer, Koenigsberg, Carr, & Appelbaum, 1989). Like an ethologist studying animal behavior, John Bowlby observed the behavior of those in attachment relationships and described what he saw. The clarity of his model provides a remarkably useful, experience-near account of abandonment and how children (and adults) respond to it. Bowlby observed toddlers separating from and returning to their mothers. He observed their behavior and emotional expression, and identified three common types of attachment: (1) *secure attachment,* in which the toddler leaves the mother, feels good alone and reunites comfortably with the mother when she returns; (2) *anxious attachment,* in which the toddler responds to the separation from the mother with definite anxiety and then clings when the mother returns; and (3) *avoidant attachment,* in which the child keeps his or her distance from the mother when she comes back into the room, as though fearful of feeling connected and then abandoned again.

Kernberg et al.'s (1989) conceptualization is based on clinical experiences with patients with borderline personality disorder, who struggle with intensely unstable interpersonal relationships and a constant fear of loss. He emphasized the aggression that is stirred up in people who are abandoned and described the terrible dilemma children have when they experience this. If their anger takes over, they feel there is no one who will take care of them and love them, so they must desperately try to reconnect with a loving object. The chaos that surrounds these patients results from their chief technique for dealing with this intense anger and loss—they try to control relationships and feelings, both internally and externally. This often involves splitting—a psychological defense where the patient separates out a good and bad self-representation and a good and bad object representation. This helps the patient maintain an inner beacon of love and hope as well as a positive feeling about others untainted by anger and hatred. Splitting maintains the inner and outer possibility of goodness. But, of course, this defensive operation causes a tremendous amount of collateral damage as well.

Many abandonment-sensitive patients have less severe symptomatology; they use more mature defenses and do not employ pathologic splitting. Bowlby's concepts of clinging attachment and avoidant attachment are helpful explanations here. This milder version of fear of abandonment looks more like a proneness to dependency. Thus, our understanding of the core problem of fear of abandonment includes those with more severe attachment problems who might have the diagnosis of borderline personality disorder as well as others with vulnerability in this area with less dysfunctional coping strategies.

The treatment goals for fear of abandonment are more stable relationships, a more consistent and integrated (good and bad) image of self and other, and less emotional reactivity (see Gunderson, 2000). In other words, the goal is to help these patients contain their destructive emotions, develop an increased ability to be effective in the world outside treatment, and increase their ability to reflect and "mentalize" (Bateman & Fonagy, 2004, 2006), that is, understand their own and others' needs and feelings.

Technique

In the treatment of a patient with fear of abandonment, there is a trend from early attention to support, behavioral control, and guidance on reasonable and healthy pragmatic choices, to a later focus on relationships and ultimately on the patient's own inner painful feelings. Gunderson's (2000) description of the stages of treatment of borderline personality disorder is clear and practical, and the stages are appropriate for the more dysfunctional patients with fear of abandonment. The initial phase is devoted to developing the treatment contract, and fleshing out this understanding usually involves some testing of the therapist. The goal is to develop the therapeutic alliance so that the feeling of consistent connection is stabilizing and does not excessively stimulate feelings of dependency and vulnerability to abandonment.

Next is a phase of relational development, which means that the patient and therapist begin to engage on a deeper, more emotional level. The intense fantasy-laden transference starts to show itself more, and the goal is to help the patient talk about it rather than act on it. Countertransferences are intense, and there is an increasing awareness of the attachment problem.

The phase of positive dependency follows and the patient begins to use other relationships to try out new self-perceptions and perceptions of others. The therapist encourages this, while helping the patient contain the intense feelings of impending loss or anger. The patient practices the ability to be connected and close to someone else, and the therapist is careful not to stimulate too much regressive dependency.

The last phase of treatment involves a more mature collaborative relationship between patient and therapist. Gunderson refers to it as an achievement of the therapeutic work that has occurred so far. The patient is now able to engage in more traditional psychodynamic insight-oriented attention to the past, present, and transference, with less of the coaching and support that has been required until now.

Another set of techniques helpful for working with patients with fear of abandonment is borrowed from mentalization-based therapy (MBT; Bateman & Fonagy, 2004, 2006) This is a psychodynamically derived treatment that frames the same process described above using somewhat different concepts and a different language. In MBT, there is a primary emphasis on the here and now with less interest in interpretation and understanding the past. Health is achieved through containment of destructive affects and increasing acceptance and awareness of emotions in the self and others. The therapist's technique focuses on helping the patient to accept and tolerate emotions, increasing his or her ability to reflect on and process them, and on avoiding interventions that stir up the patient affectively.

Transference and Countertransference

Patients with fear of abandonment often see their therapists as loving and giving, like the parental figures they longed for or, alternatively, as the worst possible version of what they experienced (e.g., as selfish, evil, dishonest, and frightening). These reactions oscillate and reflect the patient's split internal object representations. These swings are especially common in patients with more severe attachment problems. Those with less severe abandonment feel dependent on the therapist and angry about it.

Countertransference reactions are intense and can cause the therapist to express or enact feelings of powerlessness, resentment, helplessness, guilt, or defensive detachment. This is as potent a cause of compromise to the therapeutic alliance as the patient's transference reactions. The aphorism "If you don't make it worse, it will get better," captures the therapist's task well. It is our job to manage our powerful countertransference feelings, and to use them to increase our empathy and understanding of what is going on with the patient. It is easy to see how feelings are stirred up in the therapist by the patient's struggle with powerful alternating split-off experiences of merger and abandonment. Young parents of toddlers in the separation-individuation phase are confused by their children's alternating need and rejection, and the therapist with a patient who is struggling with attachment issues feels something analogous. It is not easy to maintain a healthy clinical detachment.

In our field, there can be a culture of criticizing these patients for their interpersonal dysfunction, and it is surprising how frequently trainees and faculty make derogatory jokes about patients with fear of abandonment. Of course, this distances the therapist from the patient and blames the victim. Vaillant (1992) observed that the diagnosis of borderline personality disorder can be used as an epithet and as a way of expressing unrecognized countertransference.

Low Self-Esteem

The essence of the core psychodynamic problem of low self-esteem is insecurity and loneliness that are managed through self-preoccupation and self-oriented gratification. We do not use the clinical term *narcissism* here, because that refers to a compensatory strategy used by patients with low self-esteem, rather than the problem itself, and because it has a critical and shaming connotation.

Kernberg (1975) observed that narcissistic patients show grandiose, entitled, excited, and ambitious attitudes. Different from the borderline good-and-bad self, these patients have a hugely exciting and magnificent self, along with a sad, small, depleted, shameful self. Kohut (1971, 1977, 1984) suggested a new paradigm for understanding these patients when he sensitively observed that many aggressive and entitled patients are so filled with shame, inferiority, embarrassment, and low self-esteem that virtually everything they think, feel, do, and say is directed at trying to feel better about themselves. He saw entitlement as a reaction to childhood feelings of powerlessness, loneliness, and fear, rather than a reflection of the child's anger toward frustrating parenting figures. He postulated that parents perform a "selfobject" function in early childhood, empathizing with the child's experience and providing an optimally frustrating environment that allows the child to develop the capacity to self-soothe. The selfobject function involves a balance of empathy and appropriate distance.

Developing a therapeutic alliance with patients with low self-esteem is not just the beginning of the psychotherapy, it is the essence of the treatment. Because these patients are so sensitive to criticism and rejection, building the alliance is a careful, slow process, with painstaking attention to empathy and its disruptions. Not surprisingly, given the nature of the problem, the treatment goals for patients with low self-esteem are a more reasonable and accurate self-image and the ability to tolerate vulnerability in relationships.

Technique

The psychotherapy of low self-esteem is organized around the need to support and empathize with the patient's vulnerability and easy bruisability. We watch for and deal actively with the patient's inevitable disappointment, hurt, and anger in life experiences and in the therapeutic relationship. The extensive literature on ruptures in the therapeutic alliance (e.g., Muran & Safran, 2002) suggests that although these ruptures may be inevitable in psychotherapy, they may be most problematic in patients with fragile self-esteem. If one feels insecure, one will be especially

sensitive to criticism and rejection by one's therapist. Recognizing ruptures when they occur is essential to the successful maintenance of the
alliance, and each rupture, the precipitants, the feelings stirred up by it,
and its repair are like a "teachable moment," when another empathic
building block of security and self-esteem is added.

We encourage the patient to verbalize the feelings associated with
the rupture and develop a clear chronology and picture of what happened. This awareness, along with the therapist's understanding and
empathy, will typically go a long way toward resolving the hurt. The
repeated experience of the alliance repair cycles helps the patient with
low self-esteem develop internal confidence and conviction about
the value of his or her feelings and responses and helps to build self-
esteem.

The therapist also helps patients try new skills in interpersonal relationships. Through the discussion of many current and past relationship
experiences, you will remind them of their impact on others, something
they tend not to be aware of because of their low self-esteem. You help
patients increase their social effectiveness by reminding them of what is
really happening in an interaction from both sides and support them in
the healthy expression of their needs.

Transference and Countertransference

Kohut (1971) described the common reactions of the patient with unstable self-esteem in therapy, and suggested that these transferences help us
recognize the problem. The "mirror transference" refers to the intense
need for admiration, empathy, and attention that is a replay of old needs
that went unfulfilled. Regarding the therapist as someone who will
unconditionally admire them is actually a rather controlling and insistent way of interacting which the patient employs to help manage painful
feelings of shame and unlovability. The second major transference reaction Kohut identified is idealization. Idealizing the therapist soothes the
patient because it evokes a feeling of being close to and part of someone
so special, loving, and wonderful.

Even though these two transference reactions are excessive in relation to adult needs, they reflect an essential aspect of the patient's psychological life and self-esteem problem. The transference reactions need
to be understood rather than corrected, and it is the therapist's job to
support these feelings, allow them to take root (as they have in so many
of the patient's other relationships), and ensure that the relationship
withstands the inevitable stress when the patient feels hurt, rejected, or
misunderstood.

The common countertransference reactions to patients with low self-esteem include the fantasy that the therapist will be the first truly good person in the patient's life and can provide the love and warmth that will make everything better. Other reactions include basking in the patient's idealization without noticing its inaccuracy! There may be boredom with material in the session as it can be so one-sided and self-focused, or resentment about feeling controlled by the patient's over-whelming need to be admired and protect him- or herself from being hurt by more direct and close interaction. If the transference and countertransference reactions are clear, and the ruptures and misunderstandings that take place can be explored and understood, these patients can greatly benefit from the treatment.

Panic Anxiety

Panic attacks are spontaneous acute paroxysms of anxiety. Physical symptoms such as shortness of breath, palpitations, sweating, and trembling may be associated with feelings of overwhelming fear, dying for air, or a sense of imminent disaster. Patients may become sensitized to the settings where the attacks occurred, with a resulting constriction in the radius of activity and the places that feel safe from panic.

Barbara Milrod and her group (Milrod et al., 1997, Busch et al., 2011) provide a psychodynamic formulation of panic disorder in which the central conflicts in panic patients revolve around separation and loss. Patients inhibit their anger about the sense of loss they experience with separation from caretakers because they fear that their complaints and demands might result in even greater loss. For neurobiologically vulnerable patients, these separations and losses, and the conflicts that surround them, result in panic attacks.

The therapeutic alliance gives panic patients an opportunity for support and serves as a buffer for the patient's marked sensitivity to separation and loss. But the alliance is also intertwined with the patient's struggle with the symptoms, and there is ambivalence about becoming dependent on the therapist—both a wish to be taken care of and dependent, and a reaction against this wish.

The goal of psychodynamic treatment for panic is to help the patient understand the conflicted feelings of dependency and resentment toward early caretakers which have heretofore largely been unconscious, and see how those patterns are repeated in their current experiences. This will help the patient's ability to manage close relationships in a more constructive and adaptive way. With increased healthy assertiveness and greater independence, the panic dynamics are evoked less by current circumstances and become less relevant, and the intensity and frequency of symptoms lessens.

Technique

The adaptation of psychodynamic therapy technique for panic anxiety is clearly described by Busch et al. (2011). They characterize the initial phase of treatment as developing a therapeutic alliance (with an awareness of the patient's tendency to become dependent) with a close attention to the panic history. The detailed exploration of panic attacks, especially their precipitants, and the associated thoughts, feelings, fears, and fantasies, both historical and current, takes center stage. Reality events and inner experiences can trigger an attack, and it is critical to start to see the patterns. The patient often begins the treatment thinking the attacks are spontaneous and random, but as treatment progresses, patients and therapists begin to recognize that the panic is part of a repetitive pattern.

In the second phase of therapy, the therapist helps the patient begin to see this recurring pattern of separation, anger, and inhibition of assertiveness that is typically triggered by the precipitants. Interpretations connecting the dots between the past and present are given for the many different experiences of panic or limited-symptom panic attacks the patient is experiencing. Over time, the patient begins to develop an appreciation for the complexity of his or her inner life and the consistent sequence of feelings evoked by separation and loss

As the treatment begins to move toward termination, the experience of separation from the therapist provides an *in vivo* opportunity to grasp the dynamics of separation, loss, anger, inhibition, and evolution of panic. The patient feels loss and anger about the end of the therapeutic relationship, and then anxiety about expressing it for fear of making things worse, and this may precipitate a panic attack. Sensitive attention to this phase helps the patient consolidate an emotional self-understanding and the precipitants to panic. This recognition of the panic dynamics in the transference allows for an intense but effective way to end the treatment.

Transference and Countertransference

The typical transference pattern of panic patients shows itself before termination. The chief fear is of separation and loss of the therapist. Feelings of closeness and feeling taken care of are prominent early in the treatment especially when a good therapeutic alliance takes hold. But rescheduled appointments, lateness, and vacations are felt keenly as separation, and the patient's proneness to loss and feeling alone makes these events especially charged and sometimes they lead to panic. Some patients avoid these painful emotions, just as they avoid situations in their lives which evoke panic. Confrontation about feelings that have been kept at bay, especially about loss and feeling angry about it, may trigger panic in sessions or just before or after. One patient had her first panic attack in a while immediately following an appointment in which she and her therapist tentatively discussed ending the treatment.

Typical countertransference reactions include the wish to take care of the patient and protect him or her from anxiety. This parental reaction helps the patient avoid feeling separation and loss, and also helps the therapist avoid memories and feelings about his or her own similar experiences. Frustration with the patient's dependency can lead to an urge to reject the patient and demand his or her greater independence. This would free the therapist from the uncomfortable demands for closeness. As the treatment draws to a close, and the patient is reacting to the separation, the therapist's countertransference is usually intensified in one or another of these directions.

Trauma

A trauma is an overwhelming event that threatens a patient's health, safety, or security, and is so upsetting that it cannot be effectively emotionally and cognitively processed. Responses to trauma include detachment from reality, dissociation, and the development of a split in the personality. The mind responds to trauma by walling it off, but since the thoughts, feelings, and fantasies associated with the trauma are separately maintained in a network of associations and memories, they inevitably leak back into awareness when the patient encounters something emotionally related to the traumatic experience (i.e., a trigger). These triggering experiences evoke a variety of reliving experiences that are the hallmarks of trauma: perceptual distortions, dreams, and flashbacks.

Traumatic experiences violate the bubble of safety in which we all live, and there is often a loss of innocence and trust. Perfectionism, avoidance, repetition of the traumatic situation, and dissociation are typical adaptations to trauma. A counterphobic reaction may also occur, and the trauma victim becomes very aggressive and fearless. Other adaptations include hopelessness and passivity.

The treatment goals for traumatized patients are empowerment and an increased healthy sense of safety and security. Traumatized people may have difficulty with setting up and maintaining healthy boundaries. This is especially true when the trauma has involved violence or sexual abuse. Learning how to distinguish between trustworthy and dangerous relationships leads to increased healthy trust and a greater ability to feel close and safe.

Development of the therapeutic alliance with traumatized patients is a continuous process because the issue of danger and mistrust will manifest itself there too. It takes quite a while for the patient to develop trust in the therapist and a belief that the therapist will safely and effectively carry out the relevant tasks and have the appropriate goals. The therapist must commit to genuineness in the relationship and not hide behind too much therapeutic neutrality nor maintain a blank screen with the patient. Traumatized patients are often concerned with what you are really thinking or feeling, or why you responded as you did. It may be difficult, especially early in treatment, to help the patient look at these feelings as transferential, that is, based on their previous traumatic scenarios. The patient may have experienced psychological manipulation, or at least dishonesty, in the past, and exploring the transference may feel unsafe and may provoke anxiety.

Technique

Judith Herman (1997) laid out a road map for treatment of trauma. It begins with education about the arc of psychotherapy for trauma—empowerment, exploration and evaluation of memories, and the use of that knowledge to inform current relationships and decisions. Cautious exploration of the present and past, with support, empathy, and the maintenance of a clear perspective, is the first phase. The therapist will likely need to affirm the view that the bad things that happened were wrong and may have produced lasting effects. That is, it is important to validate the experience of trauma that could have been previously denied.

Working through, the second phase, involves repeated discussion of the traumatic memories and how they are distorting current perceptions and driving current life situations. The patient can recover a sense of control, mastery, and confidence by making these perceptions more multidimensional and accurate and can start to make new decisions freed from repetition of the old traumatic scenarios.

The working through phase usually involves a deeper experiencing of the traumatic transferences (and countertransferences), and recognizing these perceptions and their historical basis deepens the level of trust in the therapeutic relationship. The therapy will be over when the old traumatic scenario is less powerful and the patient has a renewed feeling of self-efficacy and mastery, and these self-experiences are manifested in stronger relationships and greater engagement.

Transference and Countertransference

Transference patterns of trauma patients are often quite specific. That is, they are based on the details of the traumatic experience, and are released by trauma-specific triggers. Frequently a patient who was a victim of abuse regards the therapist as a potential abuser of some kind and brings that lack of trust to the relationship. It is not a general reaction, but will come forth when the therapist does something that reminds the patient of something in his or her history. For example, a female patient was scared each time the therapist closed the door to the office because of an overwhelming feeling that she was locked in and trapped with him. In this moment, it is inconceivable to a traumatized patient that the therapist could simply want to listen, help, try to understand, and protect the patient's privacy, and not have more selfish motivations that would lead to danger.

Patients may be vigilant because they feel the need to protect themselves. The rage trauma victims feel toward those who hurt them may be awakened in the transference, along with accompanied guilt or fear that the abuser (therapist) will retaliate in some way. This mixture of feelings reflects the bind they felt as helpless victims. Sometimes the transference is based on those who were bystanders and did not help, and the patient sees the therapist as having the bystander's betrayal, passivity, or cowardice.

Countertransference feelings are often strong as well. There are a number of common reactions:

1. You may identify particularly strongly with the patient's suffering and the overwhelming sense of hurt, fear, and rage and feel the urge to save and protect.
2. In response to the patient's passive bystander transference, you may feel like you are just not doing enough.
3. You may feel the urge to downplay the seriousness of the trauma and find yourself identifying with the perpetrator.
4. It may feel overwhelming to take in the description of what the trauma felt like, especially when hearing about recurrent traumatic experiences, and these feelings may cause a sense of helplessness and fear and perhaps a wish to not listen.
5. Lastly, there is a particular type of confusion the therapist may experience that is actually a form of countertransference. You may get confused about the patient's history, or forget what was discussed in the last session, or have trouble synthesizing your understanding of what the patient is talking about.

There are a variety of approaches to managing powerful countertransference experiences and you can learn more about this from the cases here as well as the more extended discussion about this in our first book (Summers & Barber, 2010, ch. 12).

This description of trauma completes the overview of the six core psychodynamic problems. The pragmatic psychodynamic therapist gathers data about the patient during the evaluation and early treatment, and choses the most appropriate problem to explain the patient's history, symptoms, current experience, and behavior. This understanding is the basis for the collaborative work of the therapeutic alliance.

How Do You Diagnose the Core Problem?

How do you determine which problem best characterizes an individual patient's issues? Often you can build a case for several different problems (see, e.g., Sharpless, Chapter 7, this volume), and there are several criteria for finding the best fit:

- What is the dominant, most painful feeling or symptom the patient is struggling with (e.g., does the patient complain of loss and loneliness, insecurity, sadness and depression, or panic attacks)?
- Does the core problem and the dynamics that go with that problem provide a reasonable explanation of the essential history, current problems, and the patient's troubling emotions? Is it the clearest, simplest, and most comprehensive explanation?
- Does the patient relate to this psychodynamic problem when you discuss it with him or her? Is there a glimmer of awareness that this problem helps to understand the difficulties?
- Will working on this problem open up the patient's awareness to allow him or her to make the desired changes?

These criteria help the therapist to frame the patient's problem. An open discussion with the patient about the problem, the potential goals of therapy, and the process for getting there will help to further build the alliance. The next chapter picks up with the next phase of therapy, when the alliance is already established and the therapist has an understanding of the patient's core problem. Now the tasks are to develop a more specific formulation and employ the psychodynamic strategies for facilitating change.

REFERENCES

Barber, J. P., Muran, J. C., McCarthy, K. S., & Keefe, R. J. (2013). Research on psychodynamic therapies. In M. J. Lambert (Ed.), *Bergin and Garfield's handbook of psychotherapy and behavior change* (6th ed., pp. 443–494). New York: Wiley.

Barlow, D. H. (Ed.). (2011). *The Oxford handbook of clinical psychology.* New York: Oxford University Press.

Bateman, A. W., & Fonagy, P. (2004). *Psychotherapy of borderline personality disorder: Mentalisation-based treatment.* Oxford, UK: Oxford University Press.

Bateman, A. W., & Fonagy, P. (2006). *Mentalization-based treatment for borderline personality disorder: A practical guide.* Oxford, UK: Oxford University Press.

Book, H. E. (1998). *How to practice brief psychodynamic psychotherapy: The CCRT method.* Washington, DC: American Psychological Association.
Bordin, E. S. (1979). The generalizability of the psychoanalytic concept of the working alliance. *Psychotherapy: Theory, Research and Practice, 16*(3), 252–260.
Bowlby, J. (1999). *Attachment and loss: Vol. 1. Attachment* (2nd ed.). New York: Basic Books. (Original work published 1982)
Busch, F. N., Milrod, B. L., Singer, M. B., & Aronson, A. C. (2011). *Manual of panic-focused psychodynamic psychotherapy—extended range.* New York: Taylor & Francis.
Busch, F. N., Rudden, M., & Shapiro, T. (2004). *Psychodynamic treatment of depression.* Arlington, VA: American Psychiatric Press.
Clarkin, J. F., Yeomans, F. E., & Kernberg O. F. (1999). *Psychotherapy for borderline personality.* New York: Wiley.
Fenichel, O. (1945). *The psychoanalytic theory of neurosis.* New York: Norton.
Freud, A. (1966). Obsessional neurosis: A summary of psycho-analytic views as presented at the congress. *International Journal of Psycho-Analysis, 47,* 116–122.
Freud, S. (1908). Character and anal erotism. In J. Strachey (Ed. & Trans.), *The standard edition of the complete psychological works of Sigmund Freud* (Vol. 9, pp. 167–175). London: Hogarth Press, 1959.
Freud, S. (1912). Recommendations to physicians practicing psycho-analysis. In J. Strachey (Ed. & Trans.), *The standard edition of the complete psychological works of Sigmund Freud* (Volume 12, pp. 109–120). London: Hogarth Press, 1959.
Gladwell, M. (2007). *Blink.* New York: Back Bay Books.
Greenson, R. R. (1967). *The technique and practice of psychoanalysis.* New York: International Universities Press.
Gunderson, J. G. (2000). Psychodynamic psychotherapy for borderline personality disorder. In J. G. Gunderson & G. O. Gabbard (Eds.), *Psychotherapy for personality disorders* (pp. 33–64). Washington, DC: American Psychiatric Press.
Herman, J. L. (1997). *Trauma and recovery: The aftermath of violence from domestic abuse to political terror.* New York: Basic Books.
Kernberg, O. F. (1975). *Borderline conditions and pathological narcissism.* New York: Jason Aronson.
Kernberg, O. F., Selzer, M. A., Koenigsberg, H. W., Carr, A. C., & Appelbaum, A. H. (1989). *Psychodynamic psychotherapy of borderline patients.* New York: Basic Books.
Kohut, H. (1971). *The analysis of the self.* New York: International Universities Press.
Kohut, H. (1977). *The restoration of the self.* New York: International Universities Press.
Kohut, H. (1984). *How does analysis cure?* New York: International Universities Press.
Leichsenring, F., & Leibling, E. (2007). Supportive-Expressive (SE) psychotherapy: An update. *Current Psychiatry Reviews, 3,* 57–64.

Luborsky, L. (1984). *Principles of psychoanalytic psychotherapy: A manual for supportive–expressive treatment.* New York: Basic Books.

Luborsky, L., & Crits-Christoph, P. (Eds.). (1998). *Understanding transference: The Core Conflictual Relationship Theme Method.* Washington, DC: American Psychological Association.

Milrod, B. L., Busch, F. N., Cooper, A. N., & Shapiro, T. (1997). *Manual of panic-focused psychodynamic psychotherapy.* Washington, DC: American Psychiatric Press.

Muran, J. C., & Barber, J. P. (Eds.). (2010). *The therapeutic alliance: An evidence-based approach to practice.* New York: Guilford Press.

Muran, J. C., & Safran, J. D. (2002). A relational approach to psychotherapy. In E. W. Kaslow (Ed.), *Comprehensive handbook of psychotherapy* (pp. 253–281). New York: Wiley.

Safran, J. D., Muran, J. C., & Eubacks-Carter, C. (2011). Repairing alliance ruptures. In J. C. Norcross (Ed.), *Psychotherapy relationships that work* (2nd ed., pp. 224–238). New York: Oxford University Press.

Salzman, L. (1968). *The obsessive personality: Origins, dynamics, and therapy.* New York: Science House.

Summers, R. F., & Barber, J. P. (2003). Therapeutic alliance as a measurable psychotherapy skill. *Academic Psychiatry, 27*(3), 160–165.

Summers, R. F., & Barber, J. P. (2010). *Psychodynamic therapy: A guide to evidence-based practice.* New York: Guilford Press

Vaillant, G. E. (1992). The beginning of wisdom is never calling a patient a borderline; or, the clinical management of immature defenses in the treatment of individuals with personality disorders. *Journal of Psychotherapy Practice and Research, 1,* 117–134.

World Health Organization. (2008). *The Global Burden Of Disease: 2004 Update.* Geneva, Switzerland: Author.

Zetzel, E. R. (1956). Current concepts of transference. *Journal of Abnormal and Social Psychology, 53,* 16–18.

CHAPTER 2

PRAGMATIC PSYCHODYNAMIC PSYCHOTHERAPY

Formulation, Therapeutic Change, and Termination

RICHARD F. SUMMERS
JACQUES P. BARBER

THE PSYCHODYNAMIC FORMULATION

With the alliance developing, and some degree of mutual understanding with the patient about the core problem, the treatment is fully underway. To really engage the patient, the therapist will need to have a specific picture of the patient's essential dynamics and how they have played out. The psychodynamic formulation is a condensed summary of the patient's specific symptoms, important experiences, central relationships, and seminal life events organized into a focused and clear conceptualization. The patient's life history is detailed, complex, richly textured, and highly individual, while the core psychodynamic problem is abstract and reflects a global understanding. The formulation represents an intermediate level of inference between the generality of the core problem and the uniqueness of the patient's life and experiences.

Developing the formulation is like connecting the dots: creating a coherent and sequential story of the patient's inner life and conflicts and demonstrating how they explain the major life events, relationships, crises, decisions, etc. The formulation helps anticipate the unfolding of the relationship between the therapist and the patient, and allows the therapist to think more specifically about what goals may be appropriate. Each of the cases in this book includes a psychodynamic formulation to demonstrate its essential role in structuring the treatment.

The approach to formulation we describe here is comprehensive—it comprises essential psychodynamics as well as the neurobiological, social, and systems aspects of the patient's problem. This approach requires the therapist to assess the relative importance of psychodynamic factors in relation to the other factors in the development and maintenance of the patient's condition. A certain amount of speculation and hypothesizing is unavoidable.

The formulation is a first attempt at understanding what makes the patient tick, and refining it will be a collaborative effort with the patient over the course of the therapy. The therapist may or may not write out a version of the formulation initially. It is desirable to do so because writing requires a higher level of scrutiny and self-reflection about the formulation than just thinking about it. In any case, the essence of the formulation should be discussed with the patient at the appropriate time. An important part of the work of the therapy will involve refining, changing, and revising this understanding.

It is hard to get started with a psychodynamic formulation for a new patient, but like any complex mental task, it is best accomplished by breaking it down into its parts, focusing on the completion of each component and anticipating the moment when it all comes together. We have developed a worksheet (Figure 2.1) to help organize the history of the patient (Summers & Barber, 2010). The optimal length of a formulation is 750–1,000 words, and it should be written simply and clearly, with as little jargon as possible. There must be multiple specific vignettes from the patient's life that illustrate the core problem and flesh out and demonstrate the general ideas suggested by the core problem.

The formulation is not a complete history. It may be hard to not include all of the information you gather, but the formulation is conceptualized at a higher level of inference than a history. Our format for formulation, based on Perry, Cooper, and Michels (1987) and Summers (2002), is divided into four parts and is summarized in Table 2.1. Although there is much that is unclear early in treatment, a good formulation commits to a coherent and specific way of organizing the data. The essential conceptualizations enable the therapist to explore the known and the unknown more purposefully and the formulation facilitates an engaged discussion with the patient. The therapist suggests new ways of understanding and actively listens to the patient's responses.

	Period of life					
	0–5 years old	5 years old– puberty	Adolescence	20s	30s	. . . or etc.
Seminal life events						
Key subjective experiences, psychiatric symptoms						
Neurobiological factors, syndromal pathology						
Psychodynamic themes						
Treatments and response						

FIGURE 2.1. Formulation worksheet. Adapted from Summers and Barber (2010). Copyright 2010 by The Guilford Press. Reprinted by permission.

Of course, developing a formulation will expose the therapist and the patient to the limitations of current knowledge about development, psychopathology, neurobiology, and related interactions. It is good to know your limits. However, focusing the therapy (Summers, Xuan, & Tavakoli, 2013) on a core psychodynamic problem, and creating a formulation that organizes the history, allows the therapist to direct attention to those issues that are most important, ensuring the greatest potential for therapeutic change.

There is great interest and an important developing literature on the cultural aspects of mental suffering and illness (American Psychological Association, 2002), including in DSM-5 (American Psychiatric Association, 2013; Lu & Primm, 2006). The psychodynamic formulation must reflect the patient's understanding of his or her symptoms, history and current situation, and it should be consistent with the essential meanings of that cultural context. The therapist needs to be aware of the patient's cultural environment and of his or her own cultural assumptions in diagnosing the core problem and developing the formulation (American Psychological Association, 2002; Rodriguez, Cabaniss, Arbuckle, & Oquendo, 2008).

TABLE 2.1. Comprehensive Psychodynamic Formulation

Part I: Summarizing statement (100–200 words only)

- Patient identification
- Precipitating events
- Most salient predisposing factors in the history
- Major historical events
- Extent and quality of interpersonal relationships
- Important aspects of neurobiology
- Behaviors that the formulation will attempt to explain

Part II: Description of nondynamic factors

- Current syndromal diagnosis
- Family history of psychiatric illness
- Syndromal psychiatric illness
- Temperamental factors
- Childhood psychopathology
- Subsyndromal illness
- Psychopharmacology experiences
- Other factors: medical illness, mental retardation, social deprivation, drugs/physical factors affecting the brain
- Traumatic experiences

Part III: Psychodynamic explanation of central conflicts

- Core psychodynamic problem
- Tracing of core problem and associated conflicts through personal history
- Include childhood example, major life event, recent example
- Explanation of patient's attempts to resolve this problem that have been maladaptive and adaptive
- Formulation of core problems and central conflicts using the psychodynamic models most useful for the problem
- Important conscious and unconscious wishes, motives, behavior, defenses
- Important developmental struggles
- Recurrent CCRT—optional
- Key strengths and how they have interacted with problems
- Effect of nondynamic factors in shaping psychodynamic problem via their effects on experience of self, other, and relationships
- Effect of dynamic factors on development and maintenance of syndromal illness

Part IV: Predicting responses to the therapeutic situation

- Prognosis, focusing on patient's experience of treatment
- Probable transference manifestations, expected resistances
- Personality strengths likely to be employed over course of treatment
- Probable reactions to psychopharmacological treatment

Note. Adapted from Summers (2002). Copyright 2002 by the Association for the Advancement of Psychotherapy. Adapted by permission.

CHANGE

We proposed a tripartite theory of change (Summers & Barber, 2010) that includes goals of therapy, mechanisms of change, and strategies for facilitating change. We will comment here on two of those components— the goals of therapy and the strategies for facilitating change—both of which are thoroughly exemplified in the cases in this book. The distinction between mechanisms of change and strategies for facilitating change is not immediately obvious. Mechanisms are those processes within the patient that are essential for change to take place, while strategies are the interventions a therapist employs to help the patient change. A discussion of therapeutic mechanisms is beyond the scope of this chapter (for more information, see Summers & Barber, 2010).

Goals of Therapy

Effective psychotherapy changes how patients feel and function. The debate about the efficacy of psychodynamic psychotherapy and its comparison to more symptom-based treatments often revolves around the question of whether treatment should simply remove symptoms (for an updated summary of what we know about the efficacy of dynamic therapy, see Barber, Muran, McCarthy, & Keefe, 2013). Reducing symptoms is clearly important and certainly makes an individual feel better, and psychodynamic therapy can and should do this. But psychodynamic therapy typically also has the aim of improving mental health and functioning. Should we simply take out the lesion and let the patient heal, or should we also try to promote new growth and change?

Mood, affect, cognition, and capacity for pleasure and mastery can all be positively affected by effective therapy. Change in one area can impact others. Potential domains of change include: (1) relationships and capacity for attachment and closeness; (2) cognitive ability to organize and focus; (3) flexibility and creativity in problem solving; (4) self-awareness; and (5) internalization of the "psychotherapy function," that is, the capacity to understand and consider alternatives (Knox, Goldberg, Woodhouse, & Hill, 1999).

Strategies for Facilitating Change

There are three sets of techniques we employ for bringing about these desired changes: (1) guiding emotional exploration, where the therapist helps the patient express feelings and thoughts and identify the repetitive scenarios that underlie the current problems; (2) searching for new accurate perceptions, where the patient is encouraged to compare and contrast old painful experiences with alternative views of similar current situations and develop new and more realistic perceptions of self and others; and (3) encouraging new behavioral responses, where the therapist supports the development and testing of new behavioral responses. In other words, our model does not place primacy on affect, cognition or behavior; instead, we suggest these are intertwined and mutually influence one another.

Emotional Exploration

New emotional awareness arises from exploration of the self that pushes past the bounds of what the patient knows or is comfortable with. The use of the term *exploration* implies that there is an unknown that can become known (Bion, 1967), and the therapist is both a goad and a guide in this process. The therapist's job is to find the old painful emotions the patient is struggling with and to help the patient give voice to them, experience them again and again so they lose their power, and develop an understanding of their original context and meaning.

The traditional mode of psychodynamic therapy involves letting the patient associate and talk about whatever is on his or her mind by inquiring, probing, and opening up areas of unexpressed feeling. This requires patience and empathy and a nose for where the emotion is and the willingness to experience it with the patient. Posing open-ended questions, working from the conscious surface down, noting avoidance and other defenses, and proposing possible explanations based on the formulation are the classic interventions of psychodynamic therapy (Williams, 2004). We agree with these approaches and note that it is important to maintain a tolerable level of anxiety in each session—not too much that makes the patient unable to reflect and explore, and not too little that allows him or her to rest on old defensive evasions. When the therapist successfully employs these interventions, the patient will feel some relief and distance from painful emotions.

For the therapist, it is an exciting sign of progress and intimacy when the patient's understanding deepens, and feelings not previously voiced are expressed. But this progress could also be somewhat intimidating because, at certain moments, the patient might feel overwhelmed by the intense affect that is evoked by the deepening understanding. Feeling previously sidestepped emotions, remembering disavowed thoughts, and recalling earlier troubling memories are all results of good exploratory techniques, but they may be unsettling.

Applying these techniques often increases anxiety in the moment, but remarkably, they also help make patients more comfortable as long as they are delivered in the frame of a supportive relationship. Anxiety decreases because painful emotions have a limited duration, and they tend to decrease in intensity relatively soon. The power of upsetting feelings is also diminished when they are overtly discussed with another person and when they start to make sense. There are specific supportive and self-soothing techniques the therapist can employ if the patient is overwhelmed and has difficulty managing this anxiety reaction to emotional exploration. You will see this illustrated in the cases (e.g., Schweitzer & Vann, Chapter 9, this volume).

There is a frequent discussion among psychodynamic therapists and psychoanalysts about whether one best understands what is happening in the patient from the perspective of a "one-person" or "two-person" psychology (Aron, 1996; Benjamin, 1990; Mitchell & Aron, 1999; Storolow & Atwood, 1992). This refers to the interesting and important question of whether it is possible to meaningfully focus on what is happening in the patient without including in that understanding what is happening in the therapist. Traditional psychoanalytic treatment is seen as employing a one-person psychological understanding because it regards the analyst's role as purely observing and interpreting, and has the taint of an authority relationship. Relational psychoanalysis (Mitchell, 2000; Mitchell & Aron, 1999), a more recent conceptual framework, suggests that most of what happens in therapy is co-created by the patient and the therapist and can only be understood when viewed from that perspective.

Our approach to this issue is pragmatic and we regard the therapist as uniquely able to observe, formulate, and employ strategies for promoting change. But, we also know that all therapists have unique personal histories with idiosyncrasies, biases, and intuitive responses, and there are many moments where an emphasis on the engagement, subjectivity, unique closeness, and meshing of emotions and perceptions that happens in good therapy is an essential focus of attention for both members of the therapeutic dyad.

New Perceptions

The second strategy for facilitating change is to promote a better and more realistic response to perceptions and feelings. This is done by encouraging patients to consider new perceptions of themselves and others, based more on a here-and-now, objective, and multidimensional viewpoint, rather than the old emotionally driven perspective.

The therapist encourages the patient to consider and review thoughts about significant others in the patient's life and helps to consider a variety of different ways of understanding difficult interpersonal situations. This technique often results in a discussion that feels like detective work.

There is a collaborative back-and-forth about possibilities; new ways of perceiving others are weighed and considered, accepted or rejected.

This second strategy for facilitating change helps develop the patient's skill of simultaneously perceiving the world based on the old painful scenarios, which were uncovered and reexperienced using the first technique for facilitating change, and seeing current realities in new and more helpful ways. The old scenarios and the adaptations to them, captured in the understanding of the core psychodynamic problem, are increasingly clear to patients, and they learn to sense when their reactions are part of the past. New perceptions are based on current adult realities and have a different feel to them from the old recurring perceptions. For example, a patient may learn to see his depressed mother as a thoughtful and resilient woman who struggles with a significant psychiatric illness (adult reality) rather than a demanding, angry, needy person who commands attention and requires him to provide complete attention and care (childhood perception).

Initially, when patients learn to notice the difference between their old and new perceptions, they may experience a delay between the moment when the same old feelings are triggered and their awareness of the contrast between this and the new adult perceptions they have worked to find. Thus, a patient may realize a day later that her reaction to an event was based on an old set of responses and become able to see another way to look at it. Further along in treatment, she may recognize the disparity between old and new perceptions soon after the triggering experiences, and ultimately this can become a more instantaneous mindful process (Badgio, Halperin, & Barber, 1999).

New Behavioral Responses

Traditional psychodynamic therapy does not explicitly focus on changing behavior because of the traditional assumption that a change in feelings will spontaneously trigger a change in behavior. But, this is not always the case and the third strategy for facilitating change is encouraging the patient to try new behaviors, evaluating the effects of such experimentation, and further modifying the behavioral responses. This was even recommended by Freud (see Barber & Luborsky, 1991).

With a greater awareness of and tolerance for painful feelings, and more adaptive perceptions of the repetitive troubling situations, the patient can try out new ways of behaving. These new behavioral responses employ social abilities and strengths evident in the nonconflictual areas of the patient's life. It is much easier for the patient to break old psychological habits and try something new now that there is a clearer picture of the old troublesome scenarios. Exercising the opportunity created by a strong therapeutic alliance, the therapist can gently suggest the need for new behaviors, pointing out that feeling differently only takes a person so far.

Sometimes patients come up with new behavioral responses themselves, sometimes they react to the therapist's suggestions, and often it is a collaborative process. Patients may begin to open up to new possibilities when they recognize that their new perceptions are out of synch with their behaviors. Alternative responses can then be considered and evaluated for comfort, effectiveness, and appropriateness.

When a patient tries something new, both the therapist and patient look at how it felt, what was different, how the patient perceived things differently, and how the others in the interaction responded differently. Trying something new and then evaluating the effects of such experimentation can be quite empowering for the patient. A repetitive troublesome experience that previously seemed immutable begins to feel like a problem that can be solved. Frequently, trying new behaviors further enhances patients' motivation in treatment.

A positive feedback loop results when new behaviors are effective. They are built on the patient's new sense of self—capable of change, strong, effective, and able to deal with painful emotions—and through their effectiveness they further validate the more mature and realistic aspects of the patient's perceptions and further reinforce the difference between old and new perceptions. This leads to more contemporary and realistic ideas about parents and significant others in the past, as well as the present. All of these trends result in more flexible thinking and healthier feeling, and a readiness to engage with the world in a more positive way.

TERMINATION

Ending therapy means a return to the struggles and joys of dealing with life without professional help. Life cycle issues and stresses continue, filtered through the continuing residue of a core psychodynamic problem, but hopefully the patient will have greater self-awareness, more accurate and contemporary perceptions, an improved capacity for self-reflection, more mature defenses, and greater strength. Maturation never stops and there will be challenges and conflict. Ideally, termination occurs when the patient wants it and is ready.

When is the right time to end? There are a variety of criteria for ending psychodynamic therapy in the literature, such as symptom resolution, attainment of goals, internalization of the psychotherapy function, and resolution of the transference (Weiner, 1998). The patient is the best judge of whether symptom resolution has occurred sufficiently and whether goals have been attained. The notion of internalizing the function of psychotherapy, or of the therapist, refers to the patient's capacity to continue the work of therapy alone. Can the patient continue the open self-reflection, self-questioning, and awareness of perceptions of behavior achieved during the treatment? This is important because it is not possible (nor desirable, probably) for the treatment to be so thorough that every psychological issue is taken up and worked on, and every problem anticipated. The patient should be able to function independently to manage problems and work on painful emotions.

There is always a transferential aspect to the decision to end therapy, and if enough of the criteria for termination have been met and the patient wants to go, little will be accomplished by pushing the patient to stay. Unresolved wishes and fantasies, including transference wishes, such as being cared for and protected, are ubiquitous. Our goal is not to eliminate them, but rather to help the patient get some perspective and determine how much is too much.

Positive feelings are often prominent at termination in longer-term dynamic psychotherapy (Roe, Dekel, Harel, & Fennig, 2006). Work has been done, goals are met to a reasonable extent, and the patient is preparing to leave. If the treatment has been successful, both therapist and patient feel satisfaction about their work and their relationship. But ending also stirs up painful feelings of loss, sadness, and frustration. Patients feel the loss of the special closeness with the therapist, disappointment about the degree of change (or those changes that did not happen), as well as feelings of rejection, loneliness, and the echoes of old losses and separations. These reactions are present when the treatment is interrupted by external factors, but they will also be significant when the ending is desired and planned carefully.

Psychodynamic therapy facilitates the patient's ability to experience these feelings of disappointment, limitation, sadness, and frustration, and explore them. It is part of the quest for self-understanding and is an *in vivo* opportunity to understand reactions to loss and ending, which are, after all, some of the most difficult experiences that we all have to come to terms with. Patients may be reluctant to discuss their negative feelings, because they realize that the treatment has to end eventually and may worry that expressing such feelings might interfere with the process of termination. They may also be afraid to criticize the therapist and express their disappointment or discontent with the outcome. A forced termination, where the therapist leaves, is particularly likely to stir up feelings of loss and rejection in the patient and guilt in the therapist.

We see two different useful ways of conceptualizing termination: one based on the traditional model and techniques of psychodynamic therapy, and the other based on the primary care model of medicine. The traditional model regards therapy as a definitive treatment and a finite experience. Here the task of termination is the successful ending of the relationship, with the notion that the end of therapy should have a sense of finality. The transference is a focus at the end, with the attempt to evoke and resolve these feelings in a definitive way. By contrast, the primary care model sees the work of therapy as never done, and does not try to push it to a conclusion in the middle of the game, so to speak. In this model, patients come for bursts of treatment when they are having difficulty functioning, or are falling behind in their ability to effectively manage their life demands. This may happen at multiple points throughout the life cycle. Treatment is offered when needed, and as patients begin to feel better and begin to function better, they pull away from the therapy and continue the work on their own, aware that they may come back.

Ending therapy is a particularly emotional experience for trainees. They have never done it before, and it is often forced by external circumstances, such as the cost or the patient's or the therapist's departure from the area. In training clinics, patients are often passed on from trainee to trainee, and this system confronts new therapists with patients who are sometimes more experienced than they are. Less experienced therapists may be in the difficult position of treating patients previously seen by more seasoned colleagues, whom they may know and respect. This is certainly a stressful undertaking, and understanding what is happening in the therapeutic relationship, being mindful of those feelings and their potential impact, and trying to do the best job possible is the best antidote to these anxieties.

Exploration and understanding of the ending provides the patient and the therapist with closure on a complicated experience. We know more about beginning therapy than ending it, and the two main ways of conceptualizing termination—the traditional psychodynamic model with its attempt to end the relationship to maximize patient independence, and the primary care model with its recognition of continuing life cycle development—both offer meaningful approaches to a successful ending. Reflecting on the decision to end a relationship and expressing the feelings involved is a meaningful last piece of work of the therapeutic alliance. Personal emotional reactions in the therapist are frequent during the end of treatment, and like our patients, we need to reflect on the ending of the relationship to keep ourselves open, genuine, and centered.

PRAGMATIC PSYCHODYNAMIC THERAPY AND CLINICAL CASES

The cases in this book exemplify many of the ideas described in these two overview chapters and in our prior book (Summers & Barber, 2010). You will see the patient's presenting problem, the evolution of a therapeutic alliance, the therapist's psychodynamic formulation, observations about the arc of the treatment, including use of the strategies for facilitating change, and the context and content of termination. There is a beginning, middle, and an end to these stories of therapy, even those in which the treatment ends before the work is done. It is interesting to note how many cases involve an unplanned or abrupt ending, and this reflects how frequent this is in real practice, especially in training clinics.

The therapists all try to evoke a healing process that translates anger and hurt to sadness and loss, and ultimately to love and gratitude. Each therapist reflects on the treatment and the patient's progress and some share with us personal comments and revelations along the way. We have written introductory remarks about each case to establish connections between our model and the cases and point out interesting moments and important dilemmas.

REFERENCES

American Psychiatric Association. (2013). Cultural Formulation Interview (CFI). In *Diagnostic and statistical manual of mental disorders* (5th ed., pp. 750–757). Arlington, VA: Author.

American Psychological Association. (2002). Guidelines on multicultural education, training, research, practice, and organizational change for psychologists. *American Psychologist, 58*(5), 377–402.

Aron, L. A. (1996). *A meeting of minds: Mutuality in psychoanalysis*. Hillsdale, NJ: Analytic Press.

Benjamin, J. (1990). Recognition and destruction: An outline of intersubjectivity. In L. Aron & S. A. Mitchell (Eds.), *Relational psychoanalysis: The emergence of a tradition* (Vol. 1, pp. 181–210). Hillsdale, NJ: Analytic Press.

Badgio, P. C., Halperin, G., & Barber, J. P. (1999). Acquisition of adaptive skills: Psychotherapeutic change in cognitive and dynamic therapies. *Clinical Psychology Review, 19*, 721–737.

Barber, J. P., & Luborsky, L. (1991). A psychodynamic view of simple phobias and prescriptive matching: A commentary. *Psychotherapy, 28*, 469–472.

Barber, J. P., Muran, J. C., McCarthy, K. S., & Keefe, R. J. (2013). Research on psychodynamic therapies. In M. J. Lambert (Ed.), *Bergin and Garfield's handbook of psychotherapy and behavior change* (6th ed., pp. 443–494). New York: Wiley.

Bion, W. R. (1967). *Second thoughts: Selected papers on psychoanalysis*. New York: Basic Books.

Knox, S., Goldberg, J. L., Woodhouse, S. S., & Hill, C. E. (1999). Clients' internal representations of their therapists. *Journal of Counseling Psychology, 46*, 244–256.

Lu, F., & Primm, A. (2006). Mental health disparities, diversity, and cultural competence: How psychiatry can play a role. *Academic Psychiatry, 30*, 9–15.

Mitchell, S. A. (2000). *Relationality: From attachment to intersubjectivity*. Hillsdale, NJ: Analytic Press.

Mitchell, S. A., & Aron, L. (Eds.). (1999). *Relational psychoanalysis: The emergence of a tradition*. Hillsdale, NJ: Analytic Press.

Perry, S., Cooper, A. M., & Michels, R. (1987). The psychodynamic formulation: Its purpose, structure, and clinical application. *American Journal of Psychiatry, 144*(5), 543–550.

Rodriguez, C. I., Cabaniss, C. L., Arbuckle, M. R., & Oquendo, M. A. (2008). The role of culture in psychodynamic psychotherapy: Parallel process resulting from cultural similarities between patient and therapist. *American Journal of Psychiatry, 165*, 1402–1406.

Roe, D., Dekel, R., Harel, G., & Fennig, S. (2006). Clients' reasons for terminating psychotherapy: A quantitative and qualitative inquiry. *Psychology and Psychotherapy: Theory, Research and Practice, 29*, 529–538.

Stolorow, R. D., & Atwood. G. E. (1992). *Context of being: The intersubjective foundation of psychological life*. Hillsdale, NJ: Analytic Press.

Summers, R. F. (2002). The psychodynamic formulation updated. *American Journal of Psychotherapy, 57*, 39–51.

Summers, R. F., & Barber, J. P. (2010). *Psychodynamic therapy: A guide to evidence-based practice*. New York: Guilford Press

Summers, R. F., Xuan, Y., & Tavakoli, D. T. (2013). Focus in psychotherapy: A training essential. *Psychodynamic Psychiatry, 41*, 91–110.

Weiner, I. B. (1998). *Principles of psychotherapy: Promoting evidence-based psychodynamic practice*. New York: Wiley.

Williams, N. (2004). *Psychoanalytic psychotherapy: A practitioner's guide*. New York: Guilford Press.

CHAPTER 3

PERMISSION TO TAKE A BREATH

A Case of Depression

HOLLY VALERIO

This first case history is of Carl, a man who suffered from depression, relationship problems, and difficulty pursuing his passion of writing. The chapter provides a clear description of a treatment that focuses on the replay of the patient's old conflicts with his mother and father, and how they had been getting in the way in the patient's adult life. The therapist was able to identify these conflicts collaboratively with the patient, and although there are many possible ways of framing these issues, she chose one and stuck with it. Through this consistent and firm focus, she was able to help him begin to dismantle the hard shell of emotional distance he had developed, which had kept his wife at a distance and blocked the flow of his writing. After 2 years of therapy he felt less depressed, more loving and less inhibited in his creative work. The therapy was ongoing at the time of the write up, so we do not know yet how the treatment will end.

Like many trainees and early-career therapists, the therapist in this case struggled with whether to use cognitive-behavioral therapy or psychodynamic therapy and felt some external pressure in this decision. She began cognitive therapy with the patient because this was the orientation assigned in her training clinic, but she began to notice important psychodynamic themes, especially in the patient's relationship with his wife, and also in the transference. The therapy shifted to psychodynamic therapy at the therapist's suggestion, and both patient and therapist seemed to find it deeper and more satisfying. This is probably the type of patient who would do well in any type of therapy—he is intelligent, motivated, articulate, and has considerable strengths.

The therapist has a determined but very sensitive attitude. She was able to help this angry and detached man allow himself to relax and open up, and give himself "permission to take a breath."

This chapter illustrates therapeutic change associated with a strong, well-defined, and clear psychodynamic focus, and raises interesting questions about choice of psychotherapy. Is the type of therapy that seems to feel most comfortable (and perhaps effective) a reflection of the patient's preferences and natural style of learning, or the therapist's, or both? It also raises questions about the wisdom of sequencing treatments, which seems to have worked beautifully in this case. These are difficult questions to answer with any certainty and there is not much data to help us. Nevertheless, this case illustrates the effectiveness of the therapist's flexible and nondogmatic attitude.

CHIEF COMPLAINT AND PRESENTATION

Carl was 37 years old when I began working with him. He was to become one of my cognitive therapy (CT) cases, having just completed 6 months of CT with a graduating resident. He had a history of major depressive disorder and initially presented to treatment with worsening depressive symptoms and suicidal thoughts. He expressed an interest in CT as well as pharmacological treatment at the time of intake and again during our first session together, stating he had been in "talk therapy" in the past and wanted to stick with a therapy where things were "active." I began working with him using a CT model, although from the beginning the therapy could not be described as strictly cognitive. Along the way, I sought out guidance from a psychodynamic supervisor as psychodynamic issues seemed to arise often in the treatment.

During our first session, Carl shared the details of his struggle with sadness and negativity. He described feeling that he had been on a journey back from the "abyss," a deep and lasting depression beginning nearly 10 years before. Prior to entering treatment 6 months ago with another therapist, his mood had worsened further, to the point that he was seriously contemplating suicide, a change from the constant, vague thoughts of ending his life as a "back up plan, just in case." He was a self-proclaimed pessimist and listed multiple negative thoughts that were repeat offenders in his mind. He stated that his negativity often made him feel paralyzed and led him to evaluate any progress forward as pointless. Since beginning the treatment 6 months prior, Carl had experienced substantial symptom improvement, no longer held suicide as his fated outcome, and had ended his 10-year strike against his lifelong passion, writing. Carl touched on his recent progress and described how he had been slowly coming back to life, although he did not want to be "too alive," as this seemed risky and a setup for disappointment.

One important source of Carl's recent unhappiness was his distaste for his "job," which in his opinion did not deserve to be called a "career." Over the past 3 years, he had earned his living as a car sales-man, a position which was somewhat lucrative initially. With time, he had grown to despise the practice of sales, feeling he was deceiving oth-ers in order to succeed. As a result, his effort diminished, and with it, his profits. At our first visit he spoke of car sales with an edge of dark humor, but it was clear that his view of his current employment was not a laughing matter. He longed to have his time free to focus on his writing, but repeatedly returned to the fact that bills needed to be paid, and writing and dreams were not going to meet this burden. He said his time at home was occupied by being a husband or preparing for the next day's work, but revealed that he also spent several hours each eve-ning surfing the internet and playing computer games. He hoped that therapy could aid him in being more organized and disciplined with his time management.

While his role as a husband was an important part of his identity, he added "relationship issues" to the list of things to address in therapy. He felt emotionally distant from his wife, unable to meet her needs, and frequently longed for the solitude that once provided space for his writ-ing to flourish. Carl was frustrated that he could not carve out the time needed to get his new writing project underway.

HISTORY

Carl was the only child of a brilliant but troubled mathematician and his wife, a musician with a big personality and intense emotions. Loss hit him early on, after his parents separated when he was 3 years old and his father moved out of the home. He described one of his earliest memories as standing on the stairs of his childhood home, watching his father walk out the door, and feeling that something terrible had hap-pened. Carl and his father maintained some contact, spending an occa-sional afternoon together, but these memories were fuzzy and distant. Any hope of his father returning home and his parents reuniting ended when Carl was only 8 years old.

Having waged an internal war with depression, Carl's father took his own life at age 37 without an explanation or closure for his son. Carl reacted to the news with outrage, refusing to attend the funeral and rebelling in any way he could find. Several months later, he remained angry, confused, and felt out of control. This eventually led him to believe that suicide was a potential way out whenever he "needed it." He explained in one of our early therapy sessions, "It was comforting to know that I wasn't trapped and could have some control if things went wrong." Without brothers or sisters, he was left alone with his mother, whose affection and tender emotions tended to "spill over" at times. Along with her loving displays were anxiety, neediness, and fierce anger.

School was a "good place" where Carl could be apart from his mother and work to distract himself from painful memories. He excelled academically, was well liked and popular, and found himself a star athlete on the track team. Despite his success at school, he was just a boy trying to be what his friends and teachers admired, without a sense of what he truly wanted or needed.

During high school he began to develop a sense of himself. He realized that he particularly enjoyed his English courses, and although the idea of being a writer was not necessarily what others expected, it was one that appealed to him. This interest solidified in college and he went on to pursue a Master's degree in Fine Arts at a competitive university. Carl saw his future clearly at this point. He would be a well-known author with a distinguished social network that respected his intellect and creativity.

While he did not necessarily see marriage or children in his future, he imagined being fulfilled by his career without the baggage that deep relationships could entail. This was not to say he avoided relationships with women entirely. He began dating in high school, but found these experiences riddled with stress and anxiety, analyzing any encounter for potential negative consequences that could lead to disappointment and pain. By the end of college and following several tumultuous and ultimately painful romances, he seemed to make the decision to protect himself from being hurt. He went on to enjoy a series of superficial relationships in which his partner was the one who ended up unhappy. He often chose women whom he sensed had a vicious side, allowing him to feel less guilty when he left them disappointed and alone.

Life changed for Carl when he turned 27 years old. He had been in psychotherapy intermittently for several years seeking to address the nagging feeling of self-doubt and the harsh tone of his internal monologue. He decided he was ready to face alone the emotions he had been avoiding in life and hoped it was not too late to reconnect with them. Gathering the few photos he had of himself and his father, Carl spent the next 3 days studying them, imagining the sorrow this young child must have felt when he lost his dad. Painful emotions eventually surfaced and he found himself brought to tears. Afterwards, he felt open and vulnerable and did not retreat as he had in the past.

In an interesting turn of events, it was only a few months before he met Stephanie. She was an artist, free spirited and creative in a way that made him feel understood for the first time. Carl admired her confidence and spontaneity. He did not feel cornered or pressured as he had in previous relationships, allowing his emotions to grow in their own time. Before long he found himself in love. Their first year together seemed magical and he was able to ignore the lack of real commitment between them, as well as the ex-boyfriend that she was not ready to give up on.

This was also a pivotal time for him professionally. Carl decided that his current manuscript would be his "ultimatum." Either it would be well received and he would move ahead with his dream career, or it would be a failure and he would throw in the towel. The pressure this placed on him was extreme, leading to self-doubt and procrastination. He eventually completed the project, just as a novel with a similar theme was published and gained popularity in the literary world. His hopes were crushed. At the same time, Stephanie revealed continued feelings for her ex-boyfriend and left Carl to rekindle her previous romance.

Carl often described the time that followed as the darkest period of his life. He had lost the two things he cared about most—the woman he loved and his willingness to write. This was the beginning of the depression that was still lingering when I first met him. The years in between were without effort or hope for the future. He was a man going through the motions, unconnected to the world.

He did have times when his mood would lift, for example, when he met his wife, Heather. While their relationship was growing and his emotions were deepening, Carl was also holding back, terrified of letting his guard down again. He found his way to the world of car sales, he and Heather married, and time passed. It was the approach of his own 37th birthday, perhaps reminding him of his father's suicide, that triggered the symptoms leading him to seek treatment again.

Carl's past psychiatric treatment consisted of sporadic therapy beginning at the age of 9, as well as the use of SSRI's and other antidepressants. He felt that psychotherapy had been beneficial at certain points in his life and "useless" at others. He made little mention of past therapists, and said even less about his relationships with them.

Medications for his symptoms were not without difficulties. SSRIs proved to be helpful in controlling his anxious and negative thoughts, but left him feeling "numb" and even more disconnected. He described them as making it "easier not to care." Carl had never been in a psychiatric hospital, and though suicide had been a serious consideration numerous times, he had never made an attempt. He did admit to using alcohol to "self medicate" at times. Denying that his drinking ever reached the point of being out of control, Carl described alcohol as a way to seem emotionally engaged with others without the "risk" of actually connecting. He had never made a habit of using illicit drugs, though he did experiment with marijuana in college.

CORE PSYCHODYNAMIC PROBLEM AND FORMULATION

I saw Carl as a man still struggling with the suicide of his father, the demandingness and lack of empathy of his mother, and the effects of the adaptive hard shell he had developed to deal with all of this loss. Inside he was sad and angry, but his experience was pervaded by self-criticism, shame, and failure. I saw him as suffering from the core psychodynamic problem of depression.

Using this core problem, I constructed the following psychodynamic formulation to guide treatment with Carl. I found it to be especially useful in helping me to keep dynamic themes in mind while we continued using a CT framework for the first year. As our first year of therapy came to a close, Carl and I made the decision to move to a psychodynamic model as will be described in the later section on course of treatment. The creation of a formulation early in therapy, along with occasional revisions as treatment progressed, made this a smoother transition.

Part I: Summarizing Statement

Carl is a 37-year-old male with a lifelong history of depression who has been in psychotherapy and psychiatric treatment intermittently since he was a boy. He describes a childhood rife with disappointment and pain, after losing his father to suicide at the age of 8, and a difficult relationship with his labile and often explosively angry mother who was his sole source of support. He has continued in therapy over the years to address intermittent periods of deep depression, self-doubt, and trouble with meaningful intimate relationships.

Carl describes his darkest period as beginning approximately 10 years ago, following the end of a relationship with the first woman he loved and the failed attempt to write a novel, which led him to give up on writing for close to a decade. Depressive feelings worsened as his 37th birthday approached, taking him close to suicide. With the memory of his publisher's rejection 10 years prior, he feels now that he will not be a "true writer" until he completes his current project.

Part II: Description of Nondynamic Factors

Carl carries the diagnosis of major depressive disorder, recurrent and severe, without psychotic symptoms. He has a strong family history of psychiatric illness including a father with major depressive disorder who completed suicide. In addition, Carl has a paternal cousin with depression and anxiety, and a maternal aunt with a diagnosis of alcoholism.

He suspects that his mother suffers from depression, anxiety, and borderline personality traits though she has never been formally treated or diagnosed.

He reports that temperamentally he was a child who was eager to please others and says his mother described him as a "happy baby." Carl has been treated with several psychopharmacologic regimens over the years. Currently, he appears to have responded favorably to a combination of Wellbutrin and Celexa but with the side effect of a feeling of emotional "numbness." Medically, he has remained healthy aside from occasional headaches.

Part III: Psychodynamic Explanation of Central Conflicts

Carl suffers from the core psychodynamic problem of depression. This can be understood by focusing on his salient experiences of loss as both a child and an adult. He has had limited stable positive attachments to fall back on, and he has learned through repeated disappointments that hope would always result in defeat. Carl struggles with significant feelings of self-doubt that have often caused him to meet others' expectations rather than his own.

The twin depressive dynamics of loss, anger, and guilt, as well as longing, idealization, and disappointment are present here. It is likely that Carl's self-criticism is the displacement of the anger he felt toward his parents as a child, now directed inwards where it seems more acceptable. He often discusses ways in which he "sets traps" for himself that make failure more probable, stemming from his continued self-focused anger and need to punish himself. His teenage and young adult romantic relationships were initially riddled with stress and anxiety, leading him to opt for many years of superficial connections where painful loss was impossible. His experience 10 years ago of becoming enamored with an emotionally unavailable woman, and the accompanying unrealistic and idealized expectations that he would be rescued from himself, resulted in substantial disappointment and sadness when they did not pan out.

Several events in Carl's life illustrate his core problem of depression. First, he often mentions an event that occurred at the age of 6, which he relates as traumatic and vital to understanding his relationship with his mother. He was coloring while lying on the floor of the living room and asked his mother what she thought of his artwork. She responded with fury, seeming to notice for the first time that he was there and yelling that he could mess up the carpet. He describes feeling incredibly guilty and afraid at this moment. After several minutes of rage his mother knelt down to hold him, telling him that she yelled because she loved him. Carl's memory of his mother at this young age was that she was "terrifying and so angry," but that at times she could be "warm and affectionate."

After describing this vignette, he said, "I loved her," but he also acknowledged he felt angry and betrayed by his mother, who had obviously focused on the carpet rather than him. He feared that an angry display aimed at his mother could push her away, causing her to desert him as his father had done. Likely, Carl's anger was internalized and this led him to feel shameful and unworthy of his mother's love.

Second, while the death of a parent is difficult for anyone, in Carl's case his father's death was particularly traumatic. His relationship with his father was limited because he left the home when his son was only 3 years old. Carl recalls riding his bike alongside his father and going for ice cream cones on the rare weekend day when they saw each other. Though these sparse images were remembered pleasantly, mostly Carl recalls feeling angry with his father for his absence from his life and for failing to protect him from the pain he experienced growing up.

But, he also seemed to identify with his father, as they both suffered from similar symptoms. In the act of killing himself, Carl's father effectively "gave up" on his fight with mental illness. This was interpreted as evidence that there was little hope that he himself could overcome his depressive symptoms and shortcomings and have a "normal" life. Carl's father left him without resolution or answers to his questions of why he was deserted. Just as directing anger toward his mother was impossible as a child, anger at his deceased father was unacceptable. As a result, his overwhelming feelings of loss and anger resulted in self-criticism, shame, and anger at himself.

Third, Carl's wife recently brought up the idea of taking a "romantic vacation." She showed him research she had done on the Internet, and expressed her hope that they could reconnect through time alone in an intimate setting. Carl's reaction was one of annoyance. He felt trapped and immediately restless, sure that Heather had "some issue" she wanted to work through with him on the trip. He resented the idea that he should put everything aside and go along with this "crazy idea," citing multiple reasons for its impracticality. When he expressed his views on the trip, Heather became infuriated, walking away from the dinner table and leaving the house to "get some air."

The idea of a vacation with planned time for intimacy and one-on-one conversation put Carl on guard. This type of request felt all too familiar to a man whose mother's unpredictability and poor emotional boundaries held him hostage for much of his early life. Furthermore, he doubted his ability to meet Heather's emotional needs as she requested more time and attention from him. It would be hard to stay distant from her with little distraction and the close quarters typical of a couples' retreat. He felt he would surely disappoint her once there, and refused based on his busy work schedule and financial pressure.

It is clear that Carl has a strong neurobiological predisposition toward depression. While depressed, he tended to isolate and withdraw, limiting his interactions with others who could have provided support and empathy. His interpersonal dynamics lead him to experience further loss and resentment in this setting, and this in turn triggers his biological vulnerability.

Part IV: Predicting Responses to the Therapeutic Situation

Carl's prognosis is good as evidenced by his improvement through recent therapy and medication treatment. However, there is a real likelihood that he may encounter future depressive episodes based on his long-lasting history of depression. He has developed a pattern of avoiding situations he perceives as challenging and in which there is an outcome he might care about; this may prevent potential loss and failure but it also prevents meaningful achievements. With Carl, the likely transference reaction will be feeling that the therapist is prying, attempting to draw out his vulnerabilities and set him up to be hurt. A likely resistance will be the use of superficial discourse and drawing the therapist's attention to less threatening subjects, limiting exploration of painful issues such as childhood loss.

Fortunately, Carl has many character strengths. He is creative and witty, as well as highly socially intelligent, with an innate ability to relate to those around him. These strengths, in addition to his persistence in continuing to engage in therapy, will help propel him forward in the process of bettering himself.

COURSE OF TREATMENT

Initially Carl embarked on a course of cognitive-behavioral therapy, focused on his stated treatment goals. These goals included developing a system for time management in order to keep space available for his writing, working to reframe his negative automatic thoughts about himself and the future, and improving his relationship with his wife. We met once a week, discussing these issues and employing CT strategies, such as automatic thought records and activity schedules.

Our therapeutic alliance developed naturally over time. With the directive treatment style we were engaged in, two components of the alliance were easily established: goal and task. By our third session, Carl had clearly articulated his treatment objectives. I concurred with his goals, feeling they were appropriate aims of our therapy process. He was consistently punctual, eloquently described his experiences and thoughts, and was adept at expressing insightful reflections on his behavior. The third element of the therapeutic alliance, the bond, progressed more gradually. Though he appeared to be opening up, and spoke about his thoughts in depth, I noticed that there was little talk of feelings. Even when I reviewed the thought record and asked him to describe the feeling present while various thoughts were in his mind, his answer would invariably be "numb" or "I don't know, maybe frustrated." Our discussions were populated by metaphors which were poetic and even dynamically themed, but lacked depth and specificity about him as a person. I often felt that he was creating a story, as he did in his manuscripts, which would engross and distract me and prevent me from getting too close to his pain.

The end of our first year of therapy, and my impending graduation from the residency, was a critical time. As this transition point neared, Carl and I reviewed his progress. He no longer felt depressed and was increasingly motivated to take charge of his future, having initiated a small side business. Writing at this point was on the back burner, as Carl reassured me (and himself) that when things "calmed down" he would return to the endeavor.

But, despite efforts at cognitive reframing, problem solving, and homework assignments aimed at increased connection and intimacy with his wife, he continued to feel distant and emotionally guarded with her. The question on the table was: what would Carl do next? We discussed the available options: terminating therapy, transferring to another resident to continue cognitive work, or moving to a psychodynamic model with me, as I would be staying on as a fellow.

I had decided to continue psychodynamic therapy with several of my patients following graduation and offered this option to Carl as well. Though I had often been viewing Carl's case from a psychodynamic perspective, and believed transitioning to this modality would allow for further growth particularly in his relationship with his wife, we had not discussed this thus far it therapy. He was somewhat hesitant regarding psychodynamic therapy, unsure what the difference would be based on previous experiences in "talk therapy." Weighing his options, Carl asked for more information both about the model and about my opinion.

I described the process of psychodynamic therapy, and explained that he could expect that we would delve further into his past relationships, discuss the losses he experienced and his feeling around these, and address what was happening in the room. I said that the transition could be helpful in addressing his need to maintain emotional distance in relationships and from his writing, but that ultimately I would respect and support his decision regardless of what he chose. After some contemplation, he replied, "Let's try it." Carl's decision to try a therapy model that called for letting his guard down and approaching his internal pain felt like a risk that we were accepting together. The bond between therapist and patient really began to deepen in this session.

Following the transition to dynamic therapy, our visits changed direction, with a new focus on past relationships and childhood disappointments. The first session in which Carl discussed his father was particularly interesting. He spoke of his earliest memories with him, the few that existed. What's more, he described his feelings about his father, and his longing for him to return home. He described waiting for his father to make up for his absence, and the nights he dreamt of their joyful reunion. With frequent pauses in his speech, unprecedented for him, he relayed the experience of hearing of his father's suicide. What stood out was his anger at himself. He was baffled at how he could have been so naive, "so stupid" to have hoped his father would come back. He acknowledged that his harsh judgment of his childhood self was logically unfounded, but logic did not change the emotions he felt.

Carl returned the next week, angry at himself, expressing frustration that he has been putting off writing and keeping his life on hold. The emotion he expressed was previously unheard of in our sessions together. Using Carl's core psychodynamic problem of depression, I understood that his talking about his great childhood loss, and the subsequent rage at his father who abandoned him, caused him to turn this dangerous emotion inwards where it was more tolerable. It was easier to be angry with himself for being naïve, for opening himself up to pain, and for giving up on his dreams, than to consider that at the root of his fury was fear that his father may have left because of him.

The lesson Carl carried away from this was that people leave and that you end up feeling foolish and painfully alone. This was reinforced at the age of 27 when Stephanie abandoned him. How could he trust his wife to stay? Would she also depart as soon as he exposed his vulnerability? These questions began to surface in Carl's mind now that he was opening himself up to feelings about his father.

But, Carl began working on a manuscript, his first writing project in nearly 10 years. The process was slow, as finding time to devote to the endeavor was compromised by the duties required by his "day job" and his responsibilities as a husband. He described "shutting down" any thoughts about the outcome of his work, stating that he did not want to have expectations of success. As his work progressed, Carl worried that life would soon become too busy and he would have to put the project aside. Several months later, exactly what he had predicted came to be. He offered frequent excuses to himself as to why it was not the right time to focus on writing. He sabotaged himself before his manuscript could get off the ground.

The fear of failure and disappointment that came with making an effort to achieve something paralyzed him. He vividly remembered what failure felt like and could not risk ending up there again. Combined with the frequent negative thoughts in his head about his abilities and the low likelihood of success, the only option seemed to be giving up. His internalized anger and subconscious urge to punish himself interrupted his progress, causing him to obstruct his own advancement. Ultimately, Carl began working on his writing again, but not before identifying in therapy the "trap" he had set for himself.

Carl's relationship with Heather was a frequent topic of therapy as well. At times he complained about "annoying" requests she would make, wanting him to sit in the kitchen while she cooked, or kiss her in the morning before they got out of bed. On one occasion, Heather had asked for a hug following a stressful day at work. Carl had the feeling that he had to "humor" his wife, something he was often required to do with his mother. Erratic and volatile, his mother demanded that he comply when she was in need of something, be it "crazy" or not. During this session, he described his mother's practice of singing a song each evening before going to sleep. Carl was to join her in singing "just in case something bad happened during the night." With Heather, he noted that he immediately felt "on guard" when she made requests for affection, describing that he felt "knocked off my equilibrium."

Through exploration of the recent events with his wife, as well as his memories of "humoring" his mother, Carl was able to identify his "fight, flight, or pull away" response. He saw it was triggered by something as benign as a request for a hug, was rooted in childhood issues, and was not really about Heather.

Several weeks later, he reported that he had given himself "permission" to "take a minute and breathe" when he felt cornered by Heather's requests. This allowed him to respond more appropriately. He reminded himself that his wife was not asking for something outlandish, but instead for emotional connection with her husband. Carl's frustration with his early attachments, particularly with his mother, led him to experience Heather as a stand-in for his childhood attachment figure. Learning as a boy that requests for attention and affection were the sign for impending "craziness" and the need to "pretend it's okay" had been carried over onto his wife. Carl realized that the "fragility" he sensed in his mother, and the fear that she would "lose her mind" as his father did, was inconsistent with his wife's character. This allowed him to feel more secure with his wife, particularly when it came to expressing his affection.

Carl's transference reactions were not initially what I expected for a patient with the core psychodynamic problem of depression. He did not exhibit signs of a dependent transference, desiring a close connection with the therapist in order to be taken care of or healed. In fact, the opposite pattern was observed. As described previously, Carl distanced himself from the probing eyes of the therapist. A closer connection appeared to be difficult to tolerate. There was also no overt evidence of an angry transference, and I had no sense that he saw me as critical or disappointed in him.

However, he attempted to keep me at a distance through humor and making light of serious matters, and by deflecting or depersonalizing his pain with metaphorical speech. How would it be possible for me to criticize that which I was not allowed to see? I surely would not reject someone who was likeable, humorous, and able to construct insightful and interesting reflections about the world.

His ability to keep me from getting too close, likely the fruit of years of labor in keeping his mother at arm's length, was what his wife now had to contend with in her attempts to feel connected to him. Carl and I were able to address his tendency to create distance between us in order to keep me from knowing him and possibly delivering harsh judgments. He commented that he had developed it over the years and had it "down to a science."

Though not central to our work, observing my countertransference allowed me to gain a deeper understanding of Carl. I often felt distant and separated from Carl in sessions. Frustrated by his avoidance of me, of connecting with his wife, and of facing the challenges of moving on from his existence as a car salesman, I found myself attempting to convince him to care. We often had sessions where I left feeling depleted, after spending 45 minutes encouraging him to look beyond his fear and allow himself to take risks and have hope for the future. This experience aided me in realizing his need to be pushed and cared for. Much as he denied it on the surface, some part of him wanted to be convinced that he could do better, and that there was hope for his future.

Over time, a new narrative began to take form. Carl was able to revise his picture of his life's course as one of failure and inadequacy, to one where he had survived painful losses and regained the ability to work toward a more meaningful future. Comparing his current place in the world with the fantasies he had as a teenager, Carl initially saw a man who was defeated, one who obviously lacked the talent and drive to accomplish anything worthwhile. Through exploration of his past losses, and confrontation of painful emotions, a different story took shape. Perhaps it was not a lack of potential or a fatal character flaw that led Carl to his present station in life. Instead, it was the pain of past disappointments holding him hostage.

The fact that he was emotionally distant was no longer an irreparable defect, or evidence that he was incapable of connecting to others. Instead, it was the survival strategy he used to get through his childhood; it would take work to reverse it, but it was reversible nonetheless. Furthermore, Carl saw himself as having options for the future. Perhaps he would finish his manuscript or look for a more fulfilling day job.

TERMINATION

At the time of writing this chapter, termination was not an issue Carl and I had broached. We had embarked on exploring his emotional responses to his wife, and how these were affected by old survival strategies employed with his mother. Though he had noted a change in his behavior with her, there was still quite a way to go. Forward motion on his manuscript has remained tenuous as well. Carl was writing—"showing up each day," as he said. However, distractions were numerous, and he was easily swayed by other "more important" obligations, quick to forget his affirmation that writing was what made him feel whole.

Perhaps writing was also where he could be honest and open about difficult and painful issues, but keep some distance. The therapeutic journey does not seem to me to be nearing its conclusion, and I ask Carl every few months about his feelings about therapy. Thus far, he and I have agreed therapy should continue.

ASSESSMENT OF PROGRESS

Carl's resilience and ability to appreciate dynamic themes was evident early in therapy, as he described his insightful understanding of his and others' behavior. However, the defenses he employed to keep negative emotions hidden and the therapist at arm's length created a challenge. Several types of change strategies were utilized in working with Carl. Taking in the therapist's view that he was capable and had a variety of options and opportunities in his future, Carl found himself less defeatist and less filled with self-doubt. Over time, his identification with the therapist's belief that car sales was not the only option, and that his pessimistic outlook was distorted, allowed him to hope for better.

Emotional exploration was a key component of treatment as already discussed. Carl reflexively kept painful feelings from surfacing, and after learning to control this reflex, he found these feelings to be transforming. Analysis of his defense mechanisms, including humor and creating a barrier with words, helped him to be able to tolerate and express feelings more. By evaluating past experiences with his mother and contrasting them with current interactions with his wife, Carl was able to see them as unique and unrelated, rather than spilling over into each other. This is an area where change is just beginning to take hold. Another recent change was the adoption of a new behavior—giving himself "permission to take a breath" before responding to his wife when he feels the urge to flee or pull away.

I think Carl would benefit from further embracing the experiences of loss in his past, particularly that of his relationship with Stephanie. He recently said, "I think I've held onto the pain of losing her for so long because she's alive and can know how much she hurt me. My father can never know what he did to me." He once described a fantasy of Stephanie unexpectedly showing up at his home and pleading with him to take her back, presumably echoing Carl's childhood wish for his father to validate how important he was and return home.

While he has begun to process his anger and disappointment with his father, much remains to be unearthed. As a result, Carl continues to struggle with the seemingly automatic recoil that occurs when hope enters his mind. This prevents him from imagining his current manuscript as a success, though he continues to write rather than shelve the project as he would have in the past. Periodically he feels emotionally distant from his wife, unable to let go of his fear of vulnerability. But, now he is learning to open up to her.

Naturally, I made mistakes during the therapy. On one occasion, during our early work together, I suggested Carl and Heather work on a joint automatic thought record. I conceived of this as an effort to help them connect and problem solve as a team. Unfortunately, the following week Carl described the assignment had gone awry. My limited experience and having only Carl's perspective on their marital conflicts resulted in unplanned consequences. Heather and Carl came away from the project annoyed and more frustrated with each other. We were able to process the experience when I acknowledged my mistake. It was the first opportunity to focus on the interaction in the room. The end result was to help humanize the therapist as a real person with faults, who existed as a partner in change, not as an adversary intent on exposing closely guarded secrets. It is my sense that Carl is pleased with the course of therapy thus far. At times he mentions his desire to be assigned homework as was the norm during our cognitive phase, and occasionally creates his own assignments to keep him focused between sessions.

As a newly trained therapist, I was able to explore the unique challenge of transitioning between therapeutic models midstream in my work with Carl. Creating and employing a psychodynamic formulation while engaged in CT helped make the shift, because I was able to pick up on dynamic themes and identify elements of transference in the midst of a cognitive framework. During CT, rather than strictly focusing on thought records, cognitive restructuring, and the present difficulties, I was able to hold the big picture more clearly in my mind. Carl's core conflicts and the dynamics shaping his symptoms were incorporated into my understanding of Carl as a person, allowing the psychodynamic therapy to take a running start. Although the timing of the transition was artificially induced by my graduation from residency, I feel it was what Carl needed to reconnect with his emotional world. The process was an opportunity for growth in both the patient and, frankly, for me. When first working with Carl as my assigned CT case, I did not foresee the degree of change I have now seen, nor did I anticipate the depths the treatment would go to.

CHAPTER 4

THE LONELY FRESHMAN

A Case of Depression

BIANCA PREVIDI

Julia is an 18-year-old college freshman with depression, social isolation, and self-defeating interpersonal patterns whose treatment is striking because of the progress she made in developing closer and more positive relationships. The therapist provides a detailed and personal account of her experience of closeness and connection with this patient, as well as some of her regrets about issues not fully explored.

You see here a good example of open-ended emotional exploration of the patient's feelings, relationship patterns, and early history and how these early experiences are understood as a template for her later dysfunctional behavior. A critical life event that brought great distress and catalyzed the patient's understanding of herself in relationships became a major focus of the treatment. Therapy increased her insight and self-awareness and also generated new perceptions and behaviors.

The therapist worked closely to help the patient expand her ability to tolerate affect, especially negative affect. This is often a hallmark of effective psychodynamic therapy. As this capacity increased, it is interesting that her self-critical thoughts and feelings, and self-defeating behavior, diminished.

Although the therapy had a planned termination because of the end of the therapist's training, there is a sense of incompleteness in this case. The therapist started to grasp the degree of the patient's anger and sadness, but by the time she was prepared to explore it more fully with the patient, the patient skipped a number of appointments and the academic year was over. Thus, the patient's feelings about her therapist's impending graduation, and the negative aspect of the transference, were not fully discussed. As a result, the therapist became more aware of her high expectations for the patient.

CHIEF COMPLAINT AND PRESENTATION

Julia walked into my office with a sheepish smile, making eye contact only momentarily before quickly looking away. She appeared depressed, with subdued facial expressions, slowness in her movements, and a deliberate quality to her soft, whispery speech. Her vibrant curly hair did not match her melancholy appearance.

"I have no motivation, no purpose, and I feel as though I don't belong in this school." Julia was an 18-year-old freshman attending a prestigious university with no history of psychiatric illness. She came to the university's counseling center in the fall of her freshman year just 2 weeks after moving to her dorm. She said, "I have wanted to speak to a therapist since I was 14." When I asked why she had waited, Julia said that she did not want to tell her parents she wanted treatment. "They wouldn't understand how I felt if I told them. I didn't want to worry them. My mom thinks I should pray more and that it will solve all my problems." They did not know about her visit to the counseling center.

Julia did not have a close relationship with her parents, calling little since leaving home. She had been struggling emotionally since coming to college, and did not want to worry or burden them by revealing her difficulties. She wished she did not have parents, while simultaneously expressing envy about some of her classmates' relationships with their parents.

Julia had diminished motivation, prominent guilt over her lack of motivation about school, difficulty concentrating, poor sleep, and a low mood for weeks prior to our first session. She said she felt sad more days than not since the age of 13, and had difficulty making and sustaining friendships. She constantly "digs deep" inside her own head, "overanalyzing everything." She procrastinated always and, because her college workload was greater than what she had had before, she had fallen behind in her classes. She felt guilty about being at school, and this worsened as she began to feel more behind. "This is what I'm supposed to do . . . do well in school. I'm on a scholarship and financial aid. My mom works so much to give me everything I need and this is the only thing I have to do. I'm just lazy."

Julia had difficulty enjoying life, even while out in the company of new college classmates. She began experimenting with alcohol, and while intoxicated she felt as though she was "just existing in time and space," a stark difference from her friends who appeared jovial when inebriated. Her guilt over her procrastination was much worse when she was drunk. She felt lonely, feared appearing pathetic, and worried she would ultimately be rejected by others. She said, "I think constantly about people's judgment and worry they will dislike me."

Julia had a sexual relationship with a male classmate that occurred mainly while they were drunk. She was physically attracted to him but felt he was not interested in her when they were sober. She heard from mutual friends that he said he would never date her and did not find her attractive. Julia was hurt by these comments but, nonetheless, found him charming and continued her physical relationship with him. She was drawn to him but was unable to explain why.

After three sessions, Julia asked about meeting twice a week and inquired about medications. It was clear she had been suffering from a chronic low mood for many years and from a recent worsening of neurovegetative symptoms. She met criteria for dysthymic and major depressive disorders. She was articulate, insightful, and interested in learning about herself. She said she wanted to find her passion and goal in life.

HISTORY

Julia was born to middle-class parents of Latin American descent. Her mother emigrated from South America, leaving an impoverished life to pursue better opportunities for her children. Her father left his country in order to attend college in the United States. She is the only child of her mother and father, and experienced a "sheltered suburban life," attending all-girls Catholic schools. Her stepsister, from her father's first marriage, is 17 years older and lived with them until Julia was a teenager.

She described herself as a reserved, obedient child with a close relationship with her father while growing up. He encouraged her to dream about the future, and she remembers fantasizing with him about becoming an interior designer, singer, or the President of the United States. During childhood, Julia developed a love of music, practicing and learning to play the piano. Her father often sat in the living room, listening to her play and drifting off to sleep to the calming melodies she drew out of the keys.

Their relationship dramatically changed the day her father picked her up from school while intoxicated. She was in the eighth grade, and remembers the terrifying experience of the car swerving dangerously on the way home. Upon arriving home, she was breathless and her heart was racing, and she ran into her mother's arms. This was unusual because she was not usually so affectionate with her mother. Her father's license was suspended after a subsequent incident of driving under the influence. He could no longer drive her to school or to and from her extracurricular activities. Julia had been unaware that he had had a "drinking problem" and felt betrayed by him. She was angry, lost respect for her father, and viewed him as a lazy "slacker" who never lived up to his potential.

By contrast, Julia described her mother as hard-working, self-sacrificing, and highly critical. She recalls writing a paper in the fourth grade that her mother saw at her school open house, and receiving harsh criticism for her writing skills later that evening. Most of the memories of her mother's criticism came from her adolescence. Julia was often encouraged to dance with boys at their New Year's Eve parties and when she refused she was ridiculed for being introverted. Julia remembers her mother saying she needed to lose 5 pounds during puberty. With each critique, her insecurities grew. Her mother reminded her of how hard she was working to provide for Julia's afterschool activities. She said that Julia was the only reason she was staying in the relationship with her father. Of course, she felt tremendously guilty about her mother's sacrifices.

Julia lacked a sense of belonging from early childhood. She attributed this to her stepsister's systematic ostracism. Her sister often made comments such as, "we don't have to accommodate you," and "the world doesn't revolve around you." Little time was dedicated to family activities, and even meals were rarely shared. Her parents argued often, spent little time together, and lived "like they were divorced." Each member of the family lived in different parts of the house with little interaction between them. Julia longed for closeness and intimacy with her family, but felt rejected by them instead.

Julia has had difficulty sustaining friendships and says sadly, "I have ruined all the friendships I've had." She tries to maintain friendships with one or two individuals at a time and never belongs to a clique or a group of friends. She recalled a close friendship that lasted a few years in middle school but ended after the girl confronted Julia about her sarcastic joking. She felt deeply rejected by the friend, but still wanted to continue the relationship.

Julia was a healthy child, with no major medical or psychiatric illness. She did not use alcohol or drugs prior to matriculating to college. She had no history of disordered eating, but struggled with her body image. Her father suffers from alcohol abuse and her paternal aunts are diagnosed and treated for major depressive disorder.

Julia's particular strengths include curiosity, a love of learning, and humility. She is modest and respectful; it was not difficult to admire and like her. She has a naturally inquisitive mind and is interested in learning about herself and others. This strength, however, is dampened by her depression. She is preoccupied with how people will perceive her and expects negative responses more than positive ones.

CORE PSYCHODYNAMIC PROBLEM AND FORMULATION
Part I: Summarizing Statement

Julia is an 18-year-old female in her freshman year of college who excels in her academic pursuits despite chronic feelings of loneliness and dysphoria. Her depression worsened after leaving home for college and she is consumed by anger and guilt that manifest in several self-defeating behaviors. Julia felt rejected by her critical mother and disappointed by her father after he drove intoxicated with her in the car. She displayed shyness as a child and low self-esteem as a teenager. She longs for intimacy and wants to connect with her parents; she yearns for friendships and romantic relationships but her insecurity about her ability to form deep relationships results in her distancing herself from others.

Part II: Description of Nondynamic Factors

Julia meets the diagnostic criteria of major depressive disorder. Her two paternal aunts have major depressive disorder and her father suffers from alcohol abuse with a prior DUI arrest. Julia was a shy child and an avoidant and self-critical adolescent whose mood remained chronically low throughout her teenage years. The reckless and dangerous drive home from school, which she was forced to endure with her father as he drove her home inebriated, was traumatic. She has no history of psychiatric treatment in the past.

Part III: Psychodynamic Explanation of Central Conflicts

Julia's core psychodynamic problem is depression. Her core conflict involves a deep sense of loss in her relationships with her early caregivers along with feelings of sadness and aloneness, leading to anger toward her mother and father. She turns the anger against herself because she feels afraid that the anger will drive them away and because she fears she has hurt them and feels guilty. The guilt manifests itself as self-critical thoughts and feelings and also as self-defeating behaviors. I will give several examples of this conflict throughout her life.

In the first vignette, during Julia's early childhood, her stepsister, 17 years her senior, made her feel like "an accessory in the family." Her stepsister picked her up from middle school one afternoon, and she expected to be dropped off at home, as usual, in order to finish her homework and write a paper. Instead, she made Julia run errands with her, driving all around town, including a wait while the sister received a manicure at a nearby salon, before returning home later that evening. In response to Julia's complaining, her sister replied, "We don't have to accommodate you." Julia felt this meant she was not included in the "we," and was not really part of the family. This intense rejection, one of many such interactions with her stepsister, caused Julia hurt and loss, but also anger. She was consumed with angry thoughts and could not express them because she felt so guilty.

Julia recalled her early teenage years as the most difficult time in her life. The second illustrative vignette is the drunken drive with her father. She recalls feeling intense fear, worrying they would crash while he swerved from side to side, sharply flinging the car around turns. She was relieved to finally reach home and cried in her mother's arms, desperately hoping to feel safe and secure. Julia felt betrayed by her father and responded by emotionally distancing herself from him. Their long talks about the details of her life stopped, and she no longer looked for his support or encouragement. When he asked for a kiss, "un besito," while tapping his cheek, she now turned her back and refused. In fact, she became profoundly angry at him, acting out this anger by disrespectfully rebuffing his entreaties, insinuating he was lazy and "a slacker," and sometimes directly telling him just that. Her anger was overwhelming and she felt guilty in turn. The guilt was expressed in a stream of self-critical comments, such as "I ruin every relationship I touch . . . I'm so messed up." She tried to "push that feeling down" and seldom called him after leaving for college.

The third vignette is about the development of Julia's current depression. Her loneliness and chronic dysphoria progressed into major depressive disorder when she left home and entered college. Although she had few relationships prior to moving away, she now felt she was completely alone. She broke up with her high school boyfriend, whom she had dated for 2 years, and parted ways with her best friend who left to attend a college outside of the Philadelphia area. The transition to college, relocation to a new city, and subsequent separation from her parents, boyfriend, and friendships was a major loss. However, she denied caring about leaving her home, asserting instead that she never really felt much for her boyfriend, and she minimized the difficulty of attending a separate college from her best friend. During the first few weeks of her first semester, Julia struggled to make friends, angry at how hard it was, blaming herself for the feelings of loneliness she had. The isolation reminded her of the feelings of isolation as a child, the loss of her father as a caretaker, the criticism of her mother, and the lack of a relationship with her stepsister. She felt it was her fault, blaming herself, and responded with self-defeating behaviors, such as missing exams, turning her work in late, and self-critical commentary.

Julia also has considerable strengths. Despite her depression, disappointments, and losses, she continues to be curious, loves learning, and is humble. There is an interaction between Julia's biological and psycho-dynamic vulnerabilities. Her temperamental vulnerability to shyness as a child contributes to her sensitivity to rejection. This sensitivity is ampli-fied during depressive states and may cause her to further withdraw. On the other hand, Julia's wish to be loved and connected to others and her self-critical nature when rejected, predisposes her for depression. She internalizes her anger and directs it toward herself, thereby leading to further deepening of her depression.

Part IV: Predicting Responses to the Therapeutic Situation

Initially, Julia will probably feel loved and taken care of by the therapist, and her wish for connection and attachment with her parents will be displaced onto the therapist as a transference reaction. This may serve to strengthen and reinforce the initial phase of therapy.

However, guilt and anger may be replayed in treatment when she encounters the limitations of the therapist and replays the disappoint-ments she feels in others, especially her father. The positive attachment to her therapist early on in therapy might also lead to idealization of the recommendations of the therapist, including medications. However, similarly, if medications fail, the patient may feel abandoned and experi-ence her typical feelings of guilt and anger within therapy. She may begin to perceive the therapist as critical, similar to her mother, and this could lead to similar patterns of distancing and isolating herself or engaging in self-defeating behaviors. Hopefully, her determination, loyalty, and curiosity will allow her to withstand the painful emotions that may arise in therapy.

COURSE OF TREATMENT

In the initial phase of therapy, I tried to provide Julia with a supportive environment, information about depression, and I worked to promote the therapeutic alliance. The second phase of therapy involved helping her identify and understand the central patterns and typical dynam-ics that contributed to her depression and framed her narrative. This allowed her to change her perceptions of how she responded to others so that she could try to change some of the behaviors that were trouble-some to her. In the third phase of treatment, as therapy progressed, Julia began to miss more sessions. We tried to work on this, and understand what was going on, but before I realized what was happening and she was able to reflect on it, my impending graduation from residency forced termination.

Not surprisingly, treatment started quickly, as Julia felt deprived of closeness and hungry for a connection that would make her feel less alone. She was committed to learning about depression and relieved to have a concrete way of understanding the symptoms she was experiencing. I pointed out that she was blaming herself for symptoms that were known to be part of a syndrome of depression: why was she so guilty about her decreased concentration, motivation, and energy? She learned she suffered from a disease, for she had a biological vulnerability, and I gave her an educational handout about major depressive disorder to take home at the end of a session. This led Julia to inquire about medications at the beginning of the next session and also to ask about meeting twice a week. I was surprised by her interest in meeting more frequently and agreed quickly. She started taking citalopram 20 mg daily and this was later increased to 40 mg daily. The educational information she acquired during this period seemed to decrease some of the shame she experienced about her "laziness" and sadness, but she continued to feel quite depressed.

From the beginning, Julia was quite self-reflective and she took easily to the tasks of being a patient. She attended her appointments consistently, spoke openly about her thoughts and feelings, and was insightful and interested in understanding herself. I listened and tried to provide new ways of reflecting on the situations she discussed. It seemed that her initial reaction to me was that I was the nonjudgmental and open-minded mother she longed for. The bond component of the therapeutic alliance was surely built on this association, and Julia seemed to quickly feel secure and she seemed to sense my genuine caring for her. In the initial appointment, Julia said her goal was "to get all of my analyzing out," and to improve her mood.

I supported her goals, and after the third session, began to formulate more clearly in my mind her major conflicts. I brought to her attention her powerful childhood yearning for a stronger bond with her parents, her disappointment in the relationships as they were, and the connection between these feelings and her difficulties acquiring and maintaining close relationships since then. By the fourth session, we had another explicit goal. We were going to try to find the reason it was difficult for Julia to have stable close relationships that were fulfilling and in doing so, try to help her with her depression.

A couple of months into the treatment, Julia told the following story. After overhearing a student on her hall discussing his reluctance to seek help at the university counseling center where she got her therapy, she approached him and told him about her positive experience with therapy. She liked the feeling of giving emotional support to someone else who was in need, and commented, "I would be a professional friend if I could," making explicit eye contact with me as if to acknowledge she was saying something about me. During the same session, she revealed the amount of pain she had been struggling with, feeling "profound sadness" yet "holding it in." As she expressed these intense feelings to me, there was an implicit appreciation for the attention and positive regard she felt about me and the therapy. I sensed a moment of powerful connection and the feeling that time stood still. I felt both her pain and her gratitude, and I felt intimately involved. I gave her space when she commented at the end of the session, "I'm so grateful for my relationships here; I just want to cry." And she did.

In the second phase of therapy, we focused on the meaning of many current events and the key themes in her treatment that began to emerge: self-defeating behaviors and a conflict about dependency. She was quite depressed, and perhaps more so since she had left home. She talked about the many losses in her life, including her feelings about moving away from home. She was having difficulty with her academics and this confirmed her inner sense of unworthiness.

Julia had a lifelong pattern of procrastinating in completing school assignments but she was able to succeed in high school because of her intellectual gifts. She wrote papers the morning they were due and still received high marks. However, at her university, doing the bare minimum could no longer earn her high marks. She described feeling she was "sabotaging" herself. She turned in papers late and did not study for two exams, including a final, and this resulted in an "incomplete" grade for the class. Early on, she realized her grades in music would likely lead to failure, and she unsuccessfully applied to withdraw from the class after the deadline. She said she just was not able to get herself to fill out the late withdrawal application and hand it in on time. She was on an academic scholarship and received financial aid, but felt guilty about taking classes that were enjoyable, self-critical about her symptoms, and sure she did not deserve the financial assistance.

JULIA: I'm signing up for classes next semester that I like, but taking classes that I enjoy is not massively consequential or important.

THERAPIST: It's not important?

JULIA: In my life, in the past, the things that I had to do I didn't like, and the things I enjoyed were extra. But all of the classes I signed up for are things I would enjoy for myself. I don't see myself doing anything with them for a career. It's like I'm here for my own enjoyment.

THERAPIST: It seems like that's very difficult for you.

JULIA: What do you mean?

THERAPIST: To allow yourself to enjoy life or maybe to even allow yourself to succeed.

JULIA: Absolutely (*sigh*).

THERAPIST: I wonder why that is?

JULIA: Because I don't like myself. I'm sabotaging myself. I don't deserve it.

THERAPIST: It?

JULIA: Anything.

THERAPIST: Really?!

JULIA: Well, I guess I just feel guilty that I'm here on a scholarship, using someone else's money to take classes that I don't even know if I'm even going to use in the future in some career. I don't know what I want out of life. . . . I'm not like one of those people who knows that they want to be a doctor, or a lawyer, and have a house with a white-picket fence, and family with two and a half kids and a dog.

I suggested to Julia that she had a harsh conscience with constant self-criticism and that maybe it had something to do with the anger she had about her losses. I proposed that the anger at her parents about her rejections and losses, that is, her mother's criticism and father's betrayal, was partly directed at her parents, but it was also displaced and directed at herself. Her mother had stressed the importance of going to college, since Julia would be the first in her mother's side of the family to attend college, and she often stated, "I don't want to let them down." By failing out of college she would greatly disappoint and hurt them, indirectly expressing her anger at them.

The self-defeating tendencies also displayed themselves in other areas of her life. She was highly critical of herself and often made self-deprecating remarks. Her most recent love choice was a student who sounded distant, manipulative, and disrespectful. She fantasized about having a genuine committed relationship with him, idealizing him and longing for his love. But after she discovered that he was dating another girl, Julia felt painfully disappointed and questioned what qualities she lacked. Along with guilt and self-criticism, another major theme developed in the second phase of the therapy. Julia spoke about her desire to "be in a relationship," and began to see how hard it was for her to be alone.

JULIA: None of my friends will be in my classes next semester.

THERAPIST: It's hard being by yourself.

JULIA: Yeah, everything I do is solitary.

THERAPIST: Seems like there is a pattern. When you're reminded of being by yourself or alone, like when your friend left after visiting, or the guy you hooked up with began dating someone new, you feel quite sad and irritable. The classes you are struggling in are the ones you are taking by yourself.

JULIA: Wow!

THERAPIST: Something about being alone is really difficult.

JULIA: I'm extremely dependent. I feel weird about it because I was raised to be independent. I need people so much. I feel like I'm conflicted in every aspect of my life. I want someone to tell me what to do.

THERAPIST: If I were to do that, what might you want me to say?

JULIA: I don't know.

THERAPIST: If it were your best friend?

JULIA: Study hard, don't go out, take the test, then sleep. I need someone to help motivate me.

THERAPIST: You've mentioned not having that kind of motivation and support growing up.

JULIA: Yeah, my mom would preach at me, tell me what to do, and repeated over and over that I should pray more. She always said that she would be there for me if anything should happen. "I'll always be on your side." But it never felt like she was on my side.

THERAPIST: How did it feel?

JULIA: Critical . . . but I know this means she really does care.

Up until this point in therapy, Julia had described herself to be very independent, seldom relying on others for any kind of support in life. She often reacted with denial, withdrawal, and reaction formation while discussing her dependency needs or their seeming absence. She seldom contacted her parents after leaving for college and only called after they texted her and asked her to do so. She retreated from social situations and friendships and called herself a "social recluse." It appeared now that this was her way of denying her need to be loved, nurtured, and protected. During this time, she began to distance herself from me as well. Julia periodically missed appointments and any effort to explore the meaning behind these absences was met with minimal explanation or insight. I only later realized this behavior might be a way for Julia to avoid feeling close and dependent on me.

After returning from winter break, she had a panic attack with prolonged tearfulness after an argument with some friends at college when they confronted her for teasing remarks that were "too harsh." She was reminded of how she lost her best friend at the age of 13, when she "took a joke too far" and was "too harsh" to her friend. This led to the friend cutting ties with her and this loss triggered a depression that lasted several months. Julia feared the same outcome here. She would lose the friends she had newly made, and feel alone and depressed again. This new vignette confirmed my original formulation about her losses being closely associated with anger, guilt, and self-criticism.

Later, when she herself connected the expression of anger and the loss of her close relationship, Julia said, "I really beat myself up about losing my best friend." But, the pattern continued, and when she was upset about the rift with her college friends, she went to the roof of a building on campus, feeling quite despondent and crying for hours. She thought about how she "ruins everything," and eventually went to a psychiatric emergency room after the intensity of her despair led to nausea, vomiting, and more panic.

She recovered remarkably quickly after this dramatic scene and quickly reported, "I don't really regret what happened." She announced that she had learned that it is all right to feel upset at times. Although two girls especially were friends, perhaps this separation is not a profound loss, and it certainly is not like how she felt after the falling out with her best friend as a young teenager. She seemed to have a more realistic and less idealized image of her two college friends.

Julia also realized she had been critical of these friends, sabotaging the relationships as she had with her best friend in the eighth grade. It seemed that perhaps she was rejecting them unconsciously before they are able to reject her. Perhaps Julia was even "ruining" her friendships just as she was feeling more connected, possibly in an effort to deny feelings of dependency. She did, however, begin to see how this pattern of keeping people at bay was a repetition of the isolation she felt as a child, and for the first time she realized she was not a passive player in this scenario. She had a role in orchestrating these events in her present life and could effect a different outcome to her story. After an initial intense reaction to being confronted by her friends about her harshness, Julia was able to tolerate her feelings of disappointment and anger about the criticism, and eventually reconnected with the friends at school and had a more grounded relationship with them.

It was exciting to see the change that was sparked by this incident. She had gained some important insights, changed her inaccurate perceptions, and tried new behavioral responses. She started the next session by proclaiming, "Things are so much better!" As she described what she learned from the argument with her friends I could not help but feel happy for her. She spoke about her newfound love for philosophy, improvement in getting her school work accomplished, and decision to go out to clubs less often. The guilt over feeling anger lessened and she repeated, "I've learned it's OK to feel upset." Her joy filled the room and was contagious.

During this second phase of therapy, Julia began to build a narrative about herself and her life that incorporated these ideas about loss, anger, guilt, self-defeating behaviors, and dependency. She was particularly interested in identifying the life experiences that shaped her. She reflected further on her mother's criticism, her stepsister's and best friend's rejections, father's betrayal, and her move to college. She developed a deeper understanding of how these events affected her and her new view included a change in the role she played in her life. She realized she did not have to be passive, and she began to take a more proactive stance. She began to plan more, looked forward to events in the future, and developed a sense of hope she had not experienced before. This was a dramatic change from the beginning of therapy, when life happened to her and she allowed deadlines to pass her by. As this all got clearer, she began fostering relationships with friends and reconnecting with her parents. She also seemed to be very connected to me.

So, it was surprising that in the third and final phase of therapy, Julia began to miss sessions repeatedly. She was a college freshman and had missed some appointments in the early part of therapy, but the frequency increased. She typically said she had slept through her alarm or forgot she had an appointment, and sometimes offered no explanation for her behavior. She certainly denied any negative or ambivalent feelings that could be associated with her absences. I did not realize she was distancing herself from me until I took a 2-week vacation in April. From then on, she missed a number of appointments and when she did attend, she reported feeling less depressed and coping better than before I left.

At this point, I noticed a pattern to the breaks in therapy—first, the Christmas holiday and then my vacation. Both times her depression slightly worsened before our separation and then dramatically improved during the time we spent apart and thereafter. It was as if she rebelled in my absence, feeling that "I don't need you, I can do it on my own." With the missed sessions, I felt more distant from her too, but once I saw the pattern I became more enthusiastic about engaging with her. It was now clear to me that missing sessions was a way for her to avoid feeling close to me.

TERMINATION

Terminating treatment was foreseeable and inevitable since I was graduating from my residency program in June. But, the intensity of the treatment and the changes Julia was making had made it seem remote. She had started to miss more appointments, and 2 months before the end of the academic year, we began to discuss my graduation from residency. Although she avoided discussing her thoughts and feelings associated with termination during sessions, her absences spoke volumes.

She expressed a desire to continue therapy at her university counseling center. When I asked her about how she felt about ending, she denied having any, saying only "it's fine." She was using words to describe her feelings about ending the therapy that were similar to those she had used to describe her relationship with her parents and how she did not care about losing them. She realized that most patients might have a stronger reaction to ending treatment, but she could not give a reason for her lack of emotion. She knew she felt very positively toward me and felt dependent on me, but any negative emotion about ending therapy did not resonate with her. She said, "You helped me put so much together, I don't feel depressed the same way as I came in. I wish I had brought in a present."

My mistake was not bringing up the increasingly clear meaning of her missed appointments—avoidance of the loss, and probably expression of anger at me for leaving her. But unfortunately my clarity about this came only 3 weeks prior to the end of treatment. She did show up for our last two sessions, and we spoke about her continued absences. She acknowledged the possibility that something other than oversleeping and forgetting was causing her to miss sessions. I wondered aloud whether intimacy and how uncomfortable it feels to be dependent and vulnerable were part of the explanation. She neither refuted nor acknowledged that, but said, "I will have to think about that."

ASSESSMENT OF PROGRESS

After Julia had spent winter break and 4 weeks away from therapy with her family, I was surprised to see how well she had been doing during this time. She told her parents about her diagnosis of depression and treatment with psychotherapy and medications. While visiting home, she reached out to friends and spent enjoyable time with her mother, father, stepsister, and niece. She felt she was able to tolerate being open with others. A few weeks after the holidays, she stated, "If you want the world to open up to you, you have to open up to them." She saw herself during the second half of her therapy as a "different person." She had more of a desire to connect with people and made an effort to do so.

Her symptoms of depression seemed to improve over this break as well. Her depressed mood lifted and she had increased energy, motivation, and the ability to concentrate. It seemed more consistent with the time course and effects of the therapy than specifically related to the medication she had started at the beginning of the semester, but perhaps there was a positive effect of the medication as well. During the second semester of classes Julia no longer procrastinated and her school performance improved. She no longer enjoyed drinking heavily on the weekends or going out to clubs, feeling she had less need to escape her thoughts. She would rather hang out with a group of friends in the dorm and watch movies. She became more social, approaching other students in her dorm, initiating conversations and shedding her identity as a "social recluse."

So, Julia achieved substantial symptomatic and behavioral improvement over the year of therapy. I was enthralled by her capacity for insight early on, as she greatly exceeded my expectation of what an 18-year-old was capable of in an insight-oriented psychotherapy. In reflecting on the experience, I see now that I held this somewhat idealized view of her throughout treatment, and was disappointed by the end when she did not make as much progress on her relationships as I had hoped. However, her relationships did greatly improve. I realized that I tend to expect a lot and can get disappointed by others, especially those I care most about. (My awareness of this is part of why I am a strong advocate for the therapist's therapy.)

Julia did not know what to expect out of therapy. Her wishes to have someone to discuss her life with, and be understood in a nonjudgmental setting, were met early on, allowing her to explore and change her behavior. She reflected during the last few sessions, "I actually like who I am now. . . . I have goals in life, I have friends, and I have a better relationship with my parents." She acknowledged her desire to work on gaining more confidence, finding passion, and further improvement in her self-esteem. She plans on working with another therapist through her university counseling center in the fall.

CHAPTER 5

DRIFTING AWAY

A Case of Depression and Obsessionality

KEVIN McCARTHY

Patrick, a chronically depressed man with persisting self-defeating behavior, was a difficult patient to start therapy with. He was stuck in dysfunctional behavior patterns and it required considerable patience and skill for the therapist to figure out how to intervene. The core problem was depression, and the case demonstrates the value of understanding the specific details of interactions and situations that are problematic to the patient.

As the treatment progressed, there was some symptomatic relief and an improvement in functioning, and the therapist began to wonder if another core problem—obsessionality—lay at the heart of the patient's difficulties. As the patient's powerful and pervasive sense of shame became more apparent, the therapist became committed to reconceptualizing the problem. Recognizing the need to change core problems is difficult for therapists because of our vulnerability to confirmation bias. In this case, the therapist's awareness of his countertransference wish to rescue the patient led him to recognize that he was reinforcing the patient's avoidance of his feeling of shame. Here, as is often the case, when the therapist sees the patient differently and more accurately, there is an immediate sense of greater rapport, more vigor in the work, and a sense of change in the patient.

You will also notice that the issue of anger, and defending against anger, figures prominently in each of the cases so far. Anger is a universal experience and manifests in depression, where it is the stimulus for self-guilt and criticism, and in obsessionality, where it triggers inhibition.

Another interesting aspect of this treatment is the therapist's use of humor. The patient is rather rigid and inflexible at times, and tenacious in holding onto his views. At numerous points, the therapist is able to make an interpretation, or assert it more strongly, with the use of irony, which is quite consistent with the patient's own sense of humor.

CHIEF COMPLAINT AND PRESENTATION

Patrick came to me as part of his discharge plan from the inpatient unit where he had been treated several days for suicidal ideation. On the referral sheet, the psychiatrist had handwritten in the margins all sorts of praises for Patrick as a patient: "Educated! . . . Great potential for insight! . . . Excellent candidate for dynamic therapy!" As a novice therapist working in a community mental health center, these scribbles could not have excited me more. My caseload consisted of patients mostly needing supportive interventions. While my relationships and work with these individuals were meaningful, the frequent need to manage external crises often precluded the chance to examine the internal patterns that caused the patients to find themselves in these chronic situations. Patrick seemed to me a patient who could do the work of dynamic therapy and tolerate the exploration of his internal world. What was more, he was a patient referred from a psychiatrist whose opinion I greatly respected and whom I had never known to use exclamation marks in her case notes. However, as a novice therapist working in a community mental health center, I was not aware that these comments also meant: "Be prepared for some complex and difficult work!"

Patrick's main problems were a depression of 10 years and a puzzling inability to thrive since college. Sad mood, low motivation, and low energy kept him sidelined. Hypersomnia, hopelessness, and suicidal ideation served as his escape from the world. His mind, however, did not cooperate in his avoidance. Patrick was subject to intrusive rumination about daily events, churning over interactions in which he felt angry and powerless or conversations in which he felt humiliated due to his perceived lack of social skills. His rumination was often accompanied by indigestion and intense stabbing stomach pains. Patrick denied any anxiety symptoms, reasoning that he had "already failed at everything, so what is there left to worry about?" He had no history of substance abuse or more severe psychiatric disturbance.

Patrick recalled some adjustment stress in adolescence but believed he had overcome it because he "still had hope back then." He said depression became a problem for him sometime after college, and overall it had worsened as he got older and experienced more setbacks in his life. He acknowledged some minor improvements in mood with changes in life situation and in response to psychiatric medications. Patrick had been treated with several courses of antidepressant medication and stimulants in the past 6 years corresponding to periods when he had health insurance. He had been hospitalized twice for suicidal ideation, including the recent admission that brought him to treatment with me. Even after reviewing the chronicity and extent of Patrick's symptoms, I still shared the referring psychiatrist's hope that a dynamic treatment could be helpful for this patient.

HISTORY

Patrick was 30 years old when we first met. He insisted that he had had a "normal" childhood and was reluctant to discuss his developmental history. What he would disclose was that he grew up in an intact Irish-Catholic family and was the oldest of three boys. His father was a high school football coach and an administrator in the local government, and his mother was an elementary science teacher in a local parochial school. His father had died unexpectedly of pancreatic cancer 4 years earlier without ever revealing any of his symptoms to the family. Patrick's relationships with his parents were congenial and without conflict but not particularly intimate. He felt much closer to his mother, especially because she stayed at home to raise her sons. He believed his relationship with his mother became more distant when she returned to work when he was in fifth grade. Patrick's father "wanted to see him do well" but kept a quiet, observant distance from Patrick because he "didn't know what to do with" him. His father connected with others through things and activities he himself enjoyed and was good at, but had difficulty relating to others with different aptitudes. For instance, Patrick remembered at age 10 approaching his father because "it was time I learned how to throw a football." Patrick's father was surprised because he thought Patrick was not interested in football.

As a student, Patrick exhibited early promise in grade school, thanks to special attention from his mother. He continued to do "all right" in high school and college but felt that he could have done better had he received more guidance from his parents. Patrick's parents, who had a hands-off parenting style to begin with, were preoccupied at that time with his middle brother's misbehavior and drug use. He expressed some resentment toward his brother, especially in that his brother was popular whereas he was withdrawn.

Patrick attended the major public university in his state and majored in chemistry. He described himself as "middle of the pack" among his fellow majors. He had multiple long-term romantic relationships during and after college. He was married at age 26 to a woman he had dated for a couple of years. This marriage lasted a little over a year before "debt" and "strain" lead to a divorce. Patrick described having multiple friends and acquaintances in the past. There was not a high degree of intimacy in his friendships, and most of his contact with friends had been over their shared interest in playing videogames. He had not been in contact with any of them recently despite their efforts to reach out to him. He gave various reasons for avoiding them, stating that he was too embarrassed because he had not returned their communications, because they were at a different stage in their lives (they all had families), and because he "didn't know what to say about what [he] is doing with [his] life right now."

Patrick's employment history was a sore point for him but it was the topic he was most willing to talk about in therapy. Despite his college education and intellect, he had never held a job for more than a year. The jobs he had held had led him farther and farther away from his goal of being a research chemist. He had had two stints as a laboratory technician in research and development departments of major drug manufacturers, several months as a sales account manager for a chemical firm, a tour in graduate school for chemistry, and a graveyard shift position as an environmental specialist in a chemistry lab at a university. He left each position because he felt he had screwed up in some unfixable way, and he expressed certainty that if he had not left he would have been fired. It was always ambiguous whether the incidents precipitating his resignation were truly as important to others as Patrick felt them to be. In fact, he had never once been formally reprimanded or fired.

An example of his tendency to walk away from jobs occurred while Patrick was working at one of the drug manufacturers. He had been left in charge of the lab by his supervisor who took a medical leave for 2 months. He only needed to carry out the experiments currently running in the laboratory. Despite his aptitude and prior experience, Patrick felt extremely unprepared for the task. He lamented how "naïve [his] supervisor was to trust [him] with the responsibility."

At about the same time, Patrick began dating a coworker whom he considered "out of [his] league." His attention to his work suffered because he spent much of his time thinking about and communicating with this young woman. After several weeks of infatuation, she discarded Patrick to begin a relationship with another coworker, stating openly that she had found someone "better" and "who was going somewhere." Patrick became deeply depressed over the breakup and his work stress and this was compounded when his supervisor came back from leave. Patrick was convinced he "had left a mess" and sheepishly began to avoid his supervisor, even though there was little evidence that he had not performed adequately, or that his supervisor was displeased with him.

Within a few days of his supervisor's return, Patrick felt so desperate he decided to attempt suicide using over-the-counter medications. Waking the next morning to find his attempt was unsuccessful, Patrick thought "there was nothing to do but go into work." His coworkers noticed how ill he looked, and his supervisor recommended he go home early. Patrick checked himself into an inpatient psychiatric unit where he was monitored and treated for a week. He did not tell his work what he had done or where he was, but called in sick every day from the pay-phone on the hospital ward. Patrick felt he could not face his coworkers again and resigned from his position the day he was discharged. He maintained that his supervisor expected him to quit in order to "save him the trouble of firing" him.

Despite these problems keeping a position, Patrick was not unlucky in work or love. Without exception, he was always with a job and girl-friend. At the time he began therapy, he had just started a position as a clerk at a pharmacy counter and was living with a woman he had been dating for 18 months. However, the pattern was clear. He would invariably locate some error he made or some shortcoming he possessed and walk away from the situation before being exposed. He unilaterally ended his marriage due to his inability to provide the lifestyle he wanted for his wife. He dropped out of graduate school due to incomplete work in a course, despite receiving A's in his other classes. He did not return to a job after valuable materials went missing because he was sure others suspected him without cause. He avoided friendships because his life was not in the place in which he wanted it to be. This pattern of near-ing success then retreating had left him several thousands of dollars in debt, discouraged about his ability to make it in the adult world, and convinced his dreams were shattered.

CORE PSYCHODYNAMIC PROBLEM AND FORMULATION

Part I: Summarizing Statement

Patrick is a 30-year-old male with a long-standing history of depression and problems maintaining employment. His understanding of his problems was that there was a vague something he was missing that caused him not to be able to "hack it." He frequently lamented he "was not there the day that they handed out whatever it was that everyone else had that made them able to succeed." Patrick's symptoms of depression seemed to track the pattern of losses and lost opportunities in his life, namely, his depression worsened as he accumulated more losses over the past 10 years.

Part II: Description of Nondynamic Factors

Patrick endorsed criteria for a diagnosis of major depressive disorder (MDD), which appeared to emerge in early adolescence. Unfortunately, the genetic contribution to his depression could not be assessed, as Patrick's family would not speak about family problems, including any history of mental illness. Although largely treatment refractory, Patrick's symptoms did improve somewhat with antidepressant medication. Patrick's Irish-Catholic cultural identity was also a nondynamic factor that might have influenced how he related to himself and others. Whereas Patrick did not identify strongly with the positive aspects of his culture, he was conscious of the cultural messages of humility, guilt, shame, and the feeling of being the underdog. His depression might be partially maintained by his internalization of some of these messages.

Part III: Psychodynamic Explanation of Central Conflicts

At the onset of treatment, Patrick seemed to be struggling with the core psychodynamic problem of depression. There was a clear relation between the major losses and failures in his life and his mood and his low self-esteem. His contribution to this pattern was a tendency to walk away from situations in which he anticipated failure. He walked out of his marriage because he felt unable to provide financially. He left jobs that were on his career track because he felt incompetent and exposed in the eyes of others. Turning his back and leaving these situations allowed him to avoid feeling the depths of his loss, but also added to the number of losses on the "pile" and crippled him from feeling able to face and overcome adversity. I further hypothesized that Patrick's depression was introjective in nature, that is, driven more by guilt and problems with success than by a fear of interpersonal abandonment (anaclitic).

Patrick's Core Conflictual Relationship Theme (CCRT) consisted of wishing to be competent, being criticized or rejected by others, and feeling anger and guilt that he managed through the symptoms of depression. For instance, in his romantic relationship with his coworker Patrick wanted to succeed at a long-term relationship, was rejected and made to feel "less than," and instead of overtly being angry at his ex-girlfriend he became depressed.

Patrick's psychiatrist already recognized his character strength of intellect as an asset to dynamic work, but I also noted he possessed an exceptional sense of humor, with a real appreciation for irony. Both these strengths were likely to be valuable in assisting us toward these goals when the work of therapy inevitably becomes difficult.

Dynamic and nondynamic factors are likely to interact in making up how a patient responds to their environment. The long-standing, intractable nature of Patrick's depression is likely to make symptom improvement more difficult, as neurobiological changes are likely to have occurred after being depressed for such a long period. Additionally, Patrick may be more strongly rewarded by avoidance behavior due to his repeated pattern of walking away. Cultural factors also might make certain ways of perceiving himself more acceptable to Patrick, like viewing himself as a shameful person or as an underdog.

Part IV: Predicting Responses to the Therapeutic Situation

Patrick appeared both motivated and resistant to change. He scheduled and attended appointments, but could not meet consistently due to his erratic work schedule. In therapy, he was present and engaged, but was frequently skeptical of discussing certain topics important to dynamic therapy like relationships and feelings. He had a number of different treatments in the past, including several courses of pharmacotherapy and two hospitalizations. Most treatments had little effect, and Patrick worsened because he experienced them as additional failures in his life. He felt most things outside of his control and enacted this passive stance in our treatment.

My feelings toward Patrick, or my countertransference, began even before we first met with the referring psychiatrist's comments. I was excited to rescue him from the hopelessness with which he surrounded himself. His reaction to me, or his transference, was skeptical and cautious. So from the beginning we were at an impasse, with me holding a significant investment in our relationship. I felt for him; he did not have to feel. I esteemed him; he was able to feel worthless. I hoped for better for him; he hung on to his hopelessness. This dynamic even caused me to view his physical appearance differently. I perceived him to be average height; several years later he clued me in that he was significantly shorter than average.

The goals we agreed on were to keep him employed at his job for at least a year, keep him out of the hospital, and reduce his depressive symptoms. My goals, more specifically, were to further the therapeutic relationship, explore for themes of anger and loss, especially in his early experiences, and encourage the experience and expression of these feelings, which too often Patrick turned inward instead. In the therapy, I expected to look for his ambivalence about succeeding and expected that his resignations would come at times when he was feeling that he was getting ahead. I expected that Patrick would have many guilty feelings throughout the treatment and would experience resistance to improvement. I expected to identify a harsh internal critic within Patrick, possibly a representation of his father who had died. I expected to see his early school success and special attention from his mother in his family as something he felt ambivalence about or received a message that was dangerous or unacceptable.

COURSE OF TREATMENT

I will describe three phases of psychotherapy so far, as the patient is still in treatment. The first phase of support and initial insight was followed by a period of consolidation of gains and reformulation of the problem. This reconceptualization led to a middle phase of therapy with typical issues of working through and change.

The early work of therapy was slow and mostly supportive, despite the referring psychiatrist's strong endorsement of Patrick's suitability as a psychodynamic patient. The pace and work of therapy was in response to the tenuous relationship that developed between us. While the alliance felt reasonable, there was a constant danger of rupture due to differences in our starting points in the therapy. For instance, any sign of hopefulness or encouragement on my part was frequently met with skepticism from Patrick. Additionally, Patrick wished to focus in our sessions solely on external events (work stress, evening shifts, seasonal changes, medication effects). I felt it important to consider both his external and internal worlds to best understand his difficulties. This back-and-forth between us kept me cautious and powerless for fear of pushing Patrick away, even as I had a strong desire to help him.

The supportive interventions took the form of monitoring his work performance, encouraging and reminding him of his stated goals, and providing a less harsh evaluation of his mistakes, such as self-criticism for sleeping in on his days off and not accomplishing tasks he set for himself to do. I slipped into a very directive role at times, especially when Patrick was most hopeless or avoidant. Sometimes this supportive work was helpful, as it provided Patrick assistance in organizing himself when he felt too overwhelmed. More often than not, my direction was met with an increased passivity or an overt resistance, especially when I encouraged Patrick not to avoid, like working on his resume and applying for different jobs.

The content early in therapy mirrored Patrick's focus on external factors. He invariably started sessions by pronouncing that either "not much happened" since our last meeting or by reporting on a specific crisis that he experienced the previous week. A common topic was a run-in with an entitled customer. However, it was quickly apparent that Patrick became annoyed no matter how customers behaved. If they were reserved, they were contemptuous; if they made a request, they were entitled; if they were distracted, they were elitist; if they were friendly, they were condescending.

Patrick frequently ruminated over these events for the rest of his shift and well into the night, causing indigestion and stomach pain and keeping him "too wound up" for sleep. He complained about these events, but then batted away any suggestion to look for alternatives with "there is nothing to do but stand there and take it." Interestingly, when he said this I would imagine him standing up in front of me in the session defying me to challenge his hopelessness.

My first inclination was to help Patrick see his own contribution to these problematic situations. Little his customers did would be acceptable to him, and maybe he could find internal ways to respond differently to their behavior. However, looking for alternative coping strategies was met with further passivity and hopelessness. For instance, Patrick had a mental list of rules for "how people should treat others." Because he adhered to these rules, he had a difficult time understanding why others could not. He felt they were provoking righteous indignation in him and so was unwilling to consider the ways to change his reactions.

After several repetitions of this pattern in therapy, a supervisor advised me to go "with" the resistance, meaning not to try to convince him he was wrong or that there was a different way of seeing things. When he described one of these incidents, I was to simply meet him with empathy. Not having anything to push back against, Patrick became more curious as to what these interactions meant to him. We were able to identify what Patrick felt was being transgressed here, namely, that he was as good as his customers, and should be one of them instead of serving them.

Over many iterations of similar events, we finally mapped a cycle of how he processed these experiences: he came to the interaction with a "chip on his shoulder" about wanting to be recognized for his competence; became indignant at customers due to feeling "less than" and not respected; felt he had to "stand there and take it," and did just that by directing his anger inward. In expressing this, he made a looping physical gesture directed down toward his stomach, which I noted bothered him with indigestion.

I tried to encourage Patrick to fantasize about what he would like to say to a specific customer during a bad interaction. He was reluctant to do so, but finally he meekly asked the person to treat him with more respect. I asked him why he could not express his anger, even in the confines of the session. He believed anger would cause him to become disorganized and "blurt out something stupid," leaving him "flapping in the breeze." I ventured that he was fearful of the opposite, namely, that he believed his anger too effective and that it would push away those to whom he found it important to be close.

In response to this interpretation, he described an argument he had with his wife at the kitchen table in his parents' house. He recalled taking off his wedding ring in contempt and throwing it on the table. Without the dramatic flair of anger he intended, it bounced and rather pathetically landed in a dish of applesauce in front of everyone. Too embarrassed to fish it out, he stormed out of the kitchen. His mother retrieved it while doing the dishes and left it on the windowsill by the sink, where it stayed for a number of years. He marked this incident as essentially the end of his marriage, and was reminded of the ineffectiveness of his outburst when he would see the ring on the windowsill. We concluded his anger was both scary and out of control to him, the opposite of his wish for competence, and this experience proved to him that expressing anger would lead to loss. He avoided anger by directing it toward himself instead of outward. He found ways to do this by being inept or unthreatening (tossing his ring into the applesauce, blurting out unconsidered words, walking away from jobs), and becoming angry with himself instead.

Soon there was an opportunity to test this hypothesis. Patrick had refused to honor a refill order on painkillers for a customer because an insufficient period had passed since the previous order. The customer became belligerent and abusive and insisted on seeing the manager. The manager calmed the customer down by personally preparing the order. Patrick slipped out that night without addressing the manager, ruminating all the while that he would be fired the next time he went in to work. He told me he wanted to walk away, and coolly presented a number of rationalizations about why he thought this was a good idea (e.g., he was going to be fired anyway; he could not face his manager or the customer again; he could look for work more actively if unemployed).

Despite his discomfort in doing so, I encouraged Patrick to explore in more detail what happened in this vignette. Patrick was confident that he had done the right thing by refusing to serve the customer, who had had similar incidents at the pharmacy before. However, he assumed that his manager would be irritated at him for "making a mess." I noted the discrepancy between Patrick's relatively neutral evaluation of the incident and his strong expectation that he would be punished for it with termination. Patrick was surprised by this discrepancy but not moved in his belief. Knowing he would appreciate the irony, I pointed out that even though he had been thinking about the incident for 2 whole days, he still had not come up with the observation we came to with 20 minutes of talking. I suggested that his rumination served a function to stay stuck in his head and to avoid experiencing his own emotions about the event.

Patrick did not feel he was trying to avoid, and described his rumination as quite upsetting. While acknowledging his discomfort, I suggested that perhaps the worry and guilt were "safe" familiar emotions related to his depression and perhaps he was angry at the manager for overruling and embarrassing him by pandering to the customer. He might be too frightened of this anger to express it, and instead he turned it back on himself (i.e., his manager was angry with him and wanted to fire him). In this way, his anger was directed at a safer target, himself.

Patrick absorbed our conversation, as he was getting better at tolerating psychological explanations for his problems. Interestingly, instead of his typical defeatist response that there was nothing he could do but stand there and take it, he asked me, "Well, what do I do about it?" This response still reflected a certain amount of passivity and put responsibility on me to provide a solution. However, it was an indication on some level that he was thinking about his experience in a new way. I pointed out that now he was at a crossroads in his work: he could walk away as was his habit or stay and deal with his fearful feelings as was his goal for therapy.

In the next session, Patrick reported that everything was "all right" and he did not have much to discuss. He did not mention what else happened at his job. When I asked specifically, he presented it as a simple matter of fact that he went in and worked with his supervisor without incident. I compared his casual mood this week with his feelings from last session. He again downplayed the emotional aspect and minimized the impact the experience had previously. I did not push further at this point because he did not want to revisit the experience, but I did provide support for his ability to respond differently and more adaptively than before.

This first phase of therapy was followed by a period of consolidation and reformulation of the problem. After a year and a half, Patrick was still employed at the same job, complained less of depressive symptoms, and had remained out of the hospital. His depression, while still present, was less disabling, and Patrick had less worry that it would interfere with his basic job performance. Patrick also had found a combination of medications with his psychiatrist that seemed to work well for him: nortriptyline, lithium, and synthroid. Some of the supportive work in our therapy seemed to help Patrick accept the regular monitoring of the levels of these medications.

There remained periodic exacerbations of depression, generally lasting a few days in response to some event. He was a little more positive, and admitted that because he was dissatisfied with his present situation he must have hope that things could be better. He did not always admit to progress in therapy, often downplaying the significance of any changes or attributing them to medications or external factors. I found that if I was too explicit in praising his work, there was a pushback in the form of a disputation of his progress, a complaint about how there was more to do, or a minor flare-up in symptoms the next session. Even so, we had begun to disentangle the back-and-forth dynamic we had, as Patrick grew more responsible for change and I became more relaxed and playful in how I approached our sessions. For instance, I took more risks in the therapy, like offering colorful metaphors as a way to understand Patrick's situation. He teased me for how convoluted my metaphors were, but was able to add to them and use them productively in the new narrative he was building for himself.

While Patrick could discuss his understanding of his problems more deeply, he still struggled with how practically to apply the knowledge he was gaining from our sessions. Our relationship was significantly stronger at this point, and Patrick admitted to thinking about therapy in between sessions. He had satisfied his initial goals of feeling less depressed and sticking with work, but now new ones emerged. First and foremost, Patrick saw therapy, and learning about his typical patterns, as a goal in and of itself. He was more engaged in the process of therapy, and new information often emerged from the material we had reviewed before. Secondly, Patrick felt slightly more confident about his ability to change some of his major "failures." He wanted to reduce his debt and to pursue another job.

I began to notice that Patrick's problems did not exactly fit with my formulation of depression. For instance, I did not really see a harsh introject and guilt was less of a problem for Patrick than I had anticipated. He expected punishment for his shortcomings, but it was the feeling of shame and embarrassment that tortured him the most. I began to see the dynamic of oppositionalism as key to Patrick's relationships. He struggled with being in control of his life and feeling like he had lost the ability to be "adult." He reacted with shame and anger toward those who he felt controlled him or subjected him to external standards.

Therefore, I began to see Patrick's core psychodynamic problem as obsessionality. Shame, anger, control, and avoidance of affect were now the themes I was listening for. They were much closer to the surface than before as his depression subsided. Our relationship seemed to deepen, and he felt more comfortable talking about himself. Looking back over my process notes and talking with my supervisors, this conceptualization became even more apparent. So I shifted my focus to understand the experiences that made him feel the world was beyond his ability to control and the potential shame and anger he must have felt in response. His revised CCRT was: wishing to be competent, viewing others as putting unwanted expectations on him and shaming him, and feeling anger and shame that he managed by trying to control his own mind and behaviors. This CCRT was lived out in our relationship. Patrick wanted to feel competent. In turn, I felt pressured in the therapy to help him and put expectations on him to do certain activities and to improve. He felt ashamed for needing any help and angrily resisted me in order to feel more in control.

With this new understanding of the core problem, we entered a new phase. Patrick began to discuss anger much more frequently in our sessions. He revealed that much of his work life was spent "drifting away" in order not to feel anger. He would only return to the present when "threatened" with a customer. He believed that this way of dealing with anger caused him to make simple mistakes on orders, mostly unnoticeable to others. When asked what he meant by "drifting away," he reported making lists of things in his head and revising them over and over again. The content of these obsessive lists varied from daily activities to his classic videogame collection. I interpreted this pattern to Patrick as feeling angry and out of control at work because he was not at his perceived level of competence, then using these lists as a mental way of regaining a sense of control over inconsequential things. When his anger became too strong, specifically when a customer disrupted his obsessive reverie with a request, Patrick was jolted back into consciousness and left without his defense. The simple mistakes, like miscounting pills or not prioritizing an order, allowed Patrick to express his anger passively and also assured that he would not receive additional responsibilities at work that would make him feel more overwhelmed. This understanding of his obsessional thinking was built in pieces over many sessions and many repetitions of the similar events.

Patrick described these obsessional symptoms as an "alarm" that he could not turn off and that got louder and more obnoxious if he tried to ignore it. For instance, his obsessional lists created an urge to buy certain things in order to complete an arbitrary "set." He insisted that the only way to manage these symptoms was to give in to them or to engage in mental trickery (emptying his wallet before going to work; telling himself "maybe tomorrow"). These strategies were costly to Patrick, often meaning he could not buy lunch on his break. I noted that the obsessive and compulsive symptoms involved the sensation of not being able to control his own mind, and he struggled to regain control by outwitting himself and controlling his environment.

Patrick began to relate many more instances of this symptom.

Around the Christmas holiday, the pharmacy where Patrick worked became busier and his customers became more impatient. Patrick let on that the depressive symptoms this year included intrusive thoughts about household items and cooking tools and a compulsion to buy things. He gave in to his compulsions 2 days in a row, and spent a few hundred dollars on items he already had. He was disgusted with himself for his lack of self-control and hid the items from his girlfriend in shame.

I asked Patrick why his obsessive–compulsive symptoms were so bad now at that time. He mentioned that he was stressed because his sister-in-law was about to give birth, and he had been shuttling his mother back and forth to the hospital because she refused to drive in the city. I expected this situation to make him feel out of control but he admitted to the opposite. He was relieved his sister-in-law was having a baby because it took pressure off him to have children as the oldest among his brothers and cousins and also as the first to have married. He described his ambivalence about having children because he was uncertain of his ability to be a father and a provider. I wondered whether his symptom of compulsively spending money on unnecessary household items was a signal that he did not want to be responsible in the household as he felt his mother would want him to be. I noted that he worried about providing and felt pressure to become a provider. Instead, he found himself spending money he did not have, so he would not need to provide for others.

Patrick smartly retorted that if his compulsive symptoms were a sign, they were not a very good one, because they were only known to him, and more recently, to me. With the same playful snarkiness, I replied that his unconscious certainly knew its audience because few others besides him and me would appreciate the irony of him compulsively buying meat tenderizers and grilling tools in the middle of winter with 12 inches of snow on the ground. He laughed, and that helped make the insight more real. He replied with his now characteristic "Well, what do I do about it?" I pointed out that having a narrative about the possible function of a symptom makes it more predictable and understandable, so that he might have the greater opportunity to decide what responsibilities he wanted for himself.

The next week Patrick was offered a position in his pharmacy placing orders with drug suppliers. The offer was based on his supervisors' recognition of his potential and his previous experience in other jobs doing related work. It was not an increase in pay and called for him to work the evening shifts he detested, but it took him away from some of the customer contact that he had so much negative feeling toward. When the position was described to him, Patrick felt overwhelmed in the moment and "didn't know what to say" and so he "blurted out" a refusal. However, his supervisors persisted, telling him to think more about it. In session, Patrick connected this incident to other similar ones where he avoided responsibility and then felt incompetent and ashamed. I added to his observations that others were expecting more of him and he had mixed feelings about this, perhaps even anger. We did not have the time to unpack these feelings, but Patrick sheepishly admitted to me that he was actually the one who had said he would think about it, not his supervisors.

We did not meet for another 2 weeks as Patrick accepted the position and was training nearly every day for it. When he did come in, he was upset that he had made minor mistakes in counting supplies and on forms. His supervisor had reviewed the errors with him and concluded that Patrick just needed to slow down. Despite this reassuring information, Patrick reported the intrusive thought in session, "What the hell is wrong with you?" He associated to this phrase, recalling being a boy helping his father on projects, specifically standing by the fuse box tripping breakers as his father tested electric work somewhere in the house. He recalled being terrified, thinking, "I can't do this! I don't want to be responsible!" Invariably, in his reluctance and nervousness he forgot to turn off a breaker when told, leading to his father getting shocked. His father then stormed downstairs and dismissed him from the task with a gruff, "What the hell is wrong with you?" I asked him how those words made him feel in those moments. Patrick frowned but replied, "Relieved."

I related that experience back to the present situation. Patrick felt that increased responsibility was foisted on him, which heightened his uncertainty about his competence to do the job. He refused the promotion, but was ignored. His understandable mistakes in the back office were like letting himself forget to switch the breaker. In part, he was hoping to be relieved of his responsibilities as well as his anxiety about not being competent. However, the tradeoff for the mistakes was an accompanying feeling of shame and failure. Shortly after this session, Patrick began to feel more competent in his new role and ceased making similar mistakes.

New narratives began to emerge at about this point in the therapy, such as a newfound feeling of pride. For instance, Patrick's mother asked him to take a look in her basement at some boxes that he had been storing there. Patrick had been avoiding this task because he was anxious the boxes contained reminders of things from his past that would make him feel ashamed. Patrick found two things, a shoebox of exams, on all of which he had received an A+, and a few abstracts for academic chemistry publications that he had written. Patrick recalled specific memories of throwing these things out when he was living at his parents', but was surprised that he had actually not. He said, "I wasn't going to need them, especially where my life was heading."

When I asked him what else he felt about finding them, other than surprise, he minimized the experience as "interesting." I wondered whether he took any pride in these achievements. Patrick admitted that he almost did not recognize them, as they felt like someone else's because they were such high quality. He sheepishly admitted that he had taken the boxes back to his apartment because "I must have wanted them at some point at least, even though I don't have the space for them."

One day Patrick casually mentioned that he had applied for a part-time job at a science museum. I was shocked, as we had discussed applying for jobs many times during the therapy. Patrick had adamantly denied being ready and was avoidant and resentful when I pushed the agenda. I told Patrick I was proud of him, and that his efforts were a major accomplishment. Patrick stated he had sent out his resume "impulsively" and now he "regretted doing it." He launched into an intellectual discussion of whether he should have put relevant work experience first on his resume or ordered his jobs chronologically. I stopped him, and again told him I was proud. I asked him to stay with the feeling of someone being proud of him. He noted that it was very uncomfortable for him because he "didn't want to be set up for a fall." I noted that it looked like the original dynamic we had established where I felt positive and hopeful for him and he protected himself from failure with his regrets. At this point in the therapy, our relationship was strong enough to talk openly about and contrast the present with where we had initially begun. Patrick was also ready to give himself and our work together some credit. He replied, "Well, I guess I am a little proud too. I ended up doing a good enough job myself."

As Patrick began to talk about and confront that shame, he was better able to assess his abilities realistically and assess his ability to control his behavior rather than feel put upon by others. In turn, he was freer to decide what he wanted for his life, which included pursuing a semblance of the dreams he had long ago given up on as out of reach.

ASSESSMENT OF PROGRESS

The referring psychiatrist was right in her assessment that Patrick was a great individual for dynamic therapy. However, the process and outcome of the therapy was not the classical experience I as a novice therapist had expected it to be. The progress that Patrick and I made included developing a stronger therapeutic relationship; reducing Patrick's depressive symptoms and increasing his ability to manage them; satisfying his early goals to remain at a job for at least a year; uncovering and tolerating his feelings around anger, shame, and lack of control; reducing the pressure of his obsessive–compulsive tendencies; and expanding his functioning to be more congruent with his obvious talents and abilities. These achievements by no means were stunning, as Patrick is the first to mention, but their growth was steady across the therapy and resulted in his becoming a more stable and insightful person.

Currently, Patrick has continued to apply for more jobs and to truly think about what he wants for a career, not just a job, as he approaches midlife. He has begun to vacation and engage in recreational activities that he had given up. He has begun to appraise many of the beliefs he has about achievement, failure, and external standards. In doing so, he has concluded that many of these beliefs were never expressed to him nor do they seem to be the values his family wanted for him to have. Finally, other areas of his life have become a topic for discussion in the sessions. We are now talking about his relationship with his girlfriend and his wish to marry again, interactions with his family that have been satisfying, and his experience of therapy and his relationship with me. Obsessive–compulsive and depressive symptoms occasionally distress him, but he feels more in control of them and his ability to function when they occur.

These gains were much more rapid and forthcoming when Patrick and I reassessed how we understood his core conflict. A depressive core psychodynamic problem and formulation fit the data gathered in early sessions very well, but what was missing was the central experience of shame that Patrick felt and could not reveal until the middle of treatment. Misidentification of the core problems, as well as errant formulations that are built from the core problems, happens not infrequently in therapy and for many different reasons. My contribution to misidentifying the core problem was my own countertransference reaction of wanting to help. I ought to have seen that there was a dynamic in which I began to try to control him and he resisted. In part, the misidentification of the core problem was an enactment in that Patrick obscured from me his deep experience of shame because it was too painful to show. He could not tolerate talking about certain topics and dismissed them as irrelevant and useless (early history and relationships, especially). I was only too happy to follow, as I thought confrontation on these topics would lead to a rupture in the relationship which my rescue fantasy would not permit.

As case formulations guide interventions, our progress was limited early on and the therapy may not have moved along as much as it could have with "accurate" interpretations. But the case formulation was an initial starting place for treatment, and it was necessary to get started.

Also, I think it was the right formulation for the time. Depression was what Patrick came to therapy for and what he thought his problem was. The patient's understanding of his or her problems must be central to the work of therapy. Patrick also was probably not ready to discuss some of the deeper issues around shame and control at that time. Only with a stronger alliance and after many repetitions of the same problematic pattern was it possible to see Patrick's struggles more clearly.

CHAPTER 6

"SHE'S JUST TRYING TO HELP"
A Case of Obsessionality

LAUREN J. ELLIOTT

The case history of Emily, a young woman whose obsessional personality traits became a major problem after she had a baby, illustrates the degree of change that can occur in a relatively long-term treatment. Emily's 1 year of psychotherapy was enough time for her to achieve a substantial degree of insight and make some meaningful behavioral changes.

The therapist, herself a young woman, gently but firmly encouraged the patient to get in touch with, and learn to tolerate, her feelings of guilt and anger. This emotional awareness permitted the patient to see how much her anger, and the defenses against it, was affecting her relationships with her husband, baby, and parents.

There are several particularly interesting aspects of this patient's treatment. First, the therapist needed to be relentless in following up on, and repeatedly pointing out, the patient's anger and her defensive strategies for avoiding this. It took consistent focus to get to a point where she could see and fully experience her anger and acknowledge her avoidance of it. Once the patient developed insight into herself and her conflicts, she saw her parents, and her mother especially, much more clearly. Her mother was loving and involved, but quite anxious and controlling.

Second, even after Emily saw her mother's anxiety more clearly, and realized her own conflicted anger, she needed quite a bit of encouragement from the therapist to consider new ways of responding to her mother and new healthier ways of interacting with her. This active emotional exploration and encouragement for trying new behaviors are typical of effective psychotherapy for patients with obsessionality.

101

Finally, the case includes a detailed and sophisticated discussion of the typical feelings and issues emerging at termination when the therapist needs to move.

The therapist is open and self-reflective in her assessment of the treatment, trying to understand how her identification with the patient may have affected some of her perceptions and decisions. The ability to honestly reflect on one's work is an important skill as it allows us to improve and deepen our work and potentially increase our effectiveness.

CHIEF COMPLAINT AND PRESENTATION

Emily was a 29-year-old woman, who initially presented for psychiatric evaluation 6 months after giving birth to her first child, feeling overwhelmed, indecisive, inadequate, and anxious. She arrived for her first visit neatly and fashionably dressed, and appeared more composed than she said she felt.

Emily had "loved being pregnant" because it garnered her attention and did not disrupt her daily routine. Several weeks after delivery, she noted increased anxiety characterized by constant worrying about "everything" and a profound difficulty with decision making. Regardless of the issue at hand, she would get stuck; she always felt she was making the "wrong" choice and that the consequences of any decision would be dire. Similarly, at the end of each day, she relentlessly reviewed decisions in her mind and sought reassurance from her husband or her mother that she had done "the right thing." She admitted that decision making had chronically been difficult for her, but that the difficulty had become extreme during the postpartum period. She was overwhelmed easily, and overcome with thoughts of being a "bad mother."

She was also overly focused on bonding with her baby, and had nagging thoughts that her daughter liked her husband and parents more than her, which caused her to withdraw from her baby and family. She would try to interact with her daughter and engage her, but didn't get the response she had observed when her family did the same. She would then turn to her husband for support, who told her to "not try so hard" and "just be natural." She was quick to tears, crying almost daily, and had incredible difficulty concentrating on tasks at home and at her full-time job as a public relations manager for a large company. She was plagued by self-doubt, guilt, and feelings of inadequacy and had pronounced difficulty with organizational and time-management skills. She was initially reluctant to seek treatment because she saw it as a profound weakness that she could not manage on her own, but did so at the urging of her husband because she felt unhappy, burdened, and powerless.

HISTORY

Emily was raised along with her two younger brothers (2 and 4 years her junior), and painted with broad strokes the picture of an ideal childhood with loving, attentive parents. She admittedly loved hearing her parents boast about her good grades and achievements to their friends. Her mother was a social worker who had put her career on hold to stay home while Emily and her brothers were young, functioning as their primary caregiver. Her mother was opinionated, strong-willed, fretful, and had a longing to be needed by others. These qualities manifested in her relationships with her children as guilt about the personal sacrifices she had made to make them her main priority, which she disclosed to them when she felt unappreciated.

Her father was a physician and worked long hours, though he was family-oriented and had made an effort to be involved at home and in his children's extracurricular activities whenever possible. He was easygoing, blithe, and flexible, implicitly sharing his wife's opinions to avoid conflict. He was also attentive, though sometimes exaggerated and overly dramatic, as Emily witnessed more recently in his interactions with her baby.

Emily was independently driven in school, and also received a lot of praise from her parents and teachers for her academic achievements, including becoming valedictorian of her high school. She found her parents' satisfaction with her successes to be especially gratifying and motivating.

She attributed her difficulty with decision making throughout her life to always receiving unsolicited comments from her mother; she valued her mother's input so much that she never deviated from what was recommended to her. She took her mother's advice as law, and never felt strongly enough to dispute or deviate from it. She reported that her parents "felt they couldn't do enough for me and my brothers . . . that's how they showed their love for us." Her mother was exceptionally involved in her life, readily offering advice and a helping hand and taking an interest in the countless mundane details of her and her friends' lives. Her father was equally involved, but more subdued, in many ways serving as his wife's sidekick, thereby avoiding conflict.

Her family psychiatric history included clinically significant anxiety in her mother and youngest brother. She described a sense of closeness among her family members, but also noted an undercurrent of conflict-avoidance that precluded complete honesty with each other. For example, she described a recurring scenario in which her middle brother solicited candid feedback from the rest of the family about whether he looked fat. Emily assumed he knew he was indeed overweight because he repeatedly inquired about his weight. But despite the family consensus that he should lose a few pounds, his siblings and parents consistently and emphatically told him that he looked great, thereby protecting his feelings rather than giving genuine advice.

Her close girlfriends since childhood were dependable, thoughtful "superwomen," who were "high maintenance," in that they required a lot of attention and had high expectations of her commitment to them. She loved their presence in her life, but felt inundated by lengthy phone conversations, frequent and extensive e-mail exchanges, and invitations. She feared she would lose her friends if she were not dedicated and loyal in this way, which was increasingly difficult during the time she was adjusting to motherhood.

She attended college near her hometown, where she met her husband Evan, now a scientist for a pharmaceutical company. He was independent, introverted, and conscientious by nature. They quickly became confidants, and developed a romance, though they lacked a "can't-keep-my-hands-off-of-you" passion from the start. This was not Emily's first serious relationship, but Emily was Evan's first love. She grudgingly moved far away from her family while her husband earned his graduate degree, but flew home to spend weekends with her family every 3 to 4 weeks. She remarked that stretching visits out any longer than that would have been difficult for her. She recognized that she was exerting a lot of effort (and incurring a lot of expenses) traveling, but could not imagine it any other way.

Emily and her husband subsequently returned to their shared hometown after much deliberation; this was a source of conflict because of her husband's fear of boundary-less relationships with Emily's family members. Her husband's fears were well-founded, as Emily felt obligated to accept every invitation (to dinners, birthday parties, holidays, baby showers, and so forth) extended by friends or family, regardless of what she wanted. She was meticulous and preoccupied with how others perceived her. She tortured herself trying to answer questions like, "Would my best friend ever forgive my absence from her mother's fundraiser?" or "What will my parents think if we spend Thanksgiving with Evan's family instead of them?" Emily described her marriage as close, but recognized that nurturing their relationship took a backseat to fulfilling work, family, and social obligations.

She also noted that her sexual relationship with her husband was never a primary focus of their marriage because of their lack of spontaneity and Emily's elaborate bedtime grooming routine, which occupied 2 to 3 hours: showering, shaving, plucking her eyebrows and barely visible facial hairs, and brushing her teeth. She was aware that this daily ritual was unusual because her college friends had teased her about it, and her family members had told her they thought it was extreme, but their comments did not bother her enough to modify her practice. Because she found her routine embarrassing, she got anxious about houseguests and limited her overnight trips away with girlfriends. But in the comfort of her home, it was certainly and shamelessly part of her day.

She enjoyed the predictable daily life she and her husband shared and was not overly concerned with her routines or preferences, as they were built into her life and were not at odds with her husband's needs or other parts of her life. Emily and Evan were excited to start a family, and knew from observing friends' experiences that it would entail a difficult adjustment. She never anticipated, however, how life altering, and therefore distressing, having a baby would be for her.

CORE PSYCHODYNAMIC PROBLEM AND FORMULATION
Part I: Summarizing Statement

Emily was a 29-year-old new mother and full-time public relations representative with chronic anxiety and perfectionism that led to difficulty completing tasks and trouble with decision making. Her sense of inadequacy was triggered by feeling burdened, even by seemingly minor tasks. As a result, she avoided following through on decisions and responsibilities, precluding attainment of mastery or satisfaction. Over all else she valued closeness among family members, both geographically and emotionally, which greatly influenced her to make choices that aligned with her family's ideals. Her closeness to her family of origin consequently affected her relationship with her husband, because marital decisions were swayed by the potential impact on Emily's relationship with her family. She had a biological predisposition for anxiety and suffered subsyndromal symptoms since childhood, but her dysphoria and ruminative worry became especially prominent and problematic after the birth of her daughter with her difficulty adjusting to motherhood.

Part II: Description of Nondynamic Factors

Emily met the diagnostic criteria for generalized anxiety disorder, postpartum major depressive disorder, and obsessive–compulsive personality disorder. Her mother and youngest brother had anxiety disorders, for which they were treated with serotonin reuptake inhibitor antidepressants for years. Emily was an anxious child, though she did not have difficulty making and keeping friends or excelling in school. She was principled and had a strict conscience, driven by fears of not meeting expectations and disappointing others, especially her parents. She had a relatively uneventful youth, and her only notable traumatic event was the loss of her grandfather in early adulthood, which traumatized her because of her amplified need for proximity and closeness to her family. She never sought psychiatric treatment in the past, and was reluctant to do so because of her strong negative conviction that initiating psychotherapy or psychopharmacology meant she was too weak to conquer her problems unassisted.

Part III: Psychodynamic Explanation of Central Conflicts

Emily's core psychodynamic problem is obsessionality. The main conflict involves prominent guilt over feelings of aggression, resulting in the need to maintain rigid control over her emotions and relationships with others in order to protect herself from experiencing intense emotion. Her unconditional positive regard for her mother masked unconscious anger toward her for not allowing Emily to separate fully into her own person with independent wishes, opinions, and needs. Emily was barely aware of her anger at the outset of treatment, and tried hard to ward off feelings of anger when they slipped into her consciousness. She was mostly aware of her immense guilt, and her anger was kept out of conscious awareness through the use of obsessional defenses. This resulted in a conflict between wanting to be close to her mother and wanting to be a self-sufficient individual.

Three life experiences illustrate why obsessionality is Emily's core problem. First, she recalled a happy childhood in which she was a "good kid" with an innate desire to please her parents. They were not particularly strict, but she always complied with their rules without question lest she disappoint them and lose their approval. She had an isolated instance as an adolescent when she tested limits by not phoning her parents while out at a friend's house, despite knowing they expected her to. When she later returned home to find her parents worried about her, she felt anxious and guilty for disrespecting them, and swore it would never happen again. These feelings and her tendency to be overly self-critical were her way of protecting herself from experiencing anger at her parents for making her call them and for not recognizing her trustworthiness and limiting her independence. She was also defensively doing and undoing, by knowingly disobeying her parents, then apologizing profusely and accepting full responsibility for her actions to counteract her aggressive intent.

Second, given her inflexibility, it was not surprising that she had difficulty adapting to the mandatory life changes imposed by an unpredictable newborn. She was consumed by thoughts of what she "should" feel and, as a result, lost the feeling of autonomy. She also compared herself to her girlfriends who were mothers and made everything look effortless, which only reinforced Emily's lack of self-confidence. Her difficulty adjusting to her new role as a mother was also related to her incomplete developmental separation from her own mother. She put pressure on herself to be an assertive, attentive mother, but felt incapable and longed for her mother's involvement in even seemingly inconsequential decisions. Even unsolicited, her mother volunteered opinions, which Emily viewed as strict commandments; she had no way of gauging whether she agreed or disagreed, she just knew she needed to adhere to her mother's advice. For example, Emily and her husband enjoyed eating dinner and watching TV together after work, and wanted to preserve this time as much as possible after having the baby, especially because of the immense effort required to get their daughter to eat anything as she began with solid foods. When her mother found out that they waited to have dinner until after they fed their daughter and put her to bed, she voiced her disapproval and stressed the importance of eating with the baby at the table for her development. Emily was guilt-stricken because she felt she was being an inept mother, hindering her daughter's growth for her own selfish wishes; this guilt increased her anxiety about making the right choices. Concealed by this guilt was her intense anger toward her mother for undercutting her decision and not giving her the chance to choose when to make the transition to eating dinner as a family. As therapy progressed, she was better able to feel and tolerate this anger, and her guilt diminished to some extent.

Third, Emily's difficulties with decision making, taking initiative, and saying "no" were also reflected in other areas of her life. For example, after her grandfather died she agreed to put her grandmother's furniture in a storage unit for later use. Her grandparents had purchased new living room furniture just prior to her grandfather's falling ill, and although it was not Emily's particular style, she knew it would please her family if she planned to use the furniture when she and her husband upgraded from their small apartment to a house in the future. Paying for the storage unit for months on end infuriated Emily and her husband because they did not have imminent plans to move and were not especially fond of the items that were stored. Emily felt obligated to take the "generous" offer initially, as she imagined it would delight her grandmother and appease the rest of the family. Although she was angry about the steadily increasing cost of storing furniture she disliked, she intellectualized that it would be nice to have a representation of her family in her future home. She knew that she could reverse this commitment at any time, but would feel too guilty if she followed through. As a result, she continuously surrendered a monthly fee and deferred a decision (and full recognition of her anger) until the following month.

The dynamics and biological vulnerability interact here. Emily likely had a genetic vulnerability to anxiety as there was a significant family history and she certainly had an anxious temperament since childhood. Her mother's sacrificing her career and her anxiety, which was present in Emily's early developmental years, likely contributed to a pattern in which Emily considered her mother's emotional needs to be more important than her own. Emily worried about her mother and felt that she needed to take care of her. This worry may have caused her to set unreasonable standards for herself that were often unattainable, leading to guilt and self-criticism. These expectations lend themselves to rigidity and a sense of duty rather than passion and conviction. In addition, Emily's self-punishment, perceived critique from others, and efforts to protect herself from intense emotion, positive or negative, likely reinforced her innate tendency to feel depressed and anxious. Her tendency toward harsh self-criticism, rather than outwardly directed anger, diminished her self-confidence, making it more difficult to assert her independence. Her fear of destroying and losing relationships by having her own opinions created further inhibition.

Emily's intelligence, articulateness, commitment to fairness, perseverance, and friendly and outgoing nature were strengths that helped her to connect to others, maintain functionality at work, and cope with daily responsibilities despite her insecurities and self-perceived insufficiencies. These traits were also positive prognostic features for psychotherapy, despite her initial reservations about exposing herself through the therapeutic process.

Part IV: Predicting Responses to the Therapeutic Situation

Given her degree of suffering and motivation to feel more secure as a mother, Emily was eager to establish a therapeutic alliance to facilitate an increased awareness of her feelings and enhance her experience of autonomy and spontaneity. However, her need to control her own feelings and desire to be autonomous may lead her to attempt to control the therapy and therapist as well. She may do so by expressing anger and hostility toward the therapist or by talking without interruption, thereby preventing the therapist from uncovering strong emotions. Her tendency to ruminate and waver on decisions may result in testing to see whether the therapist favors one decision over another. This testing may recreate the familiar dynamic with her mother and reinforce a counterproductive battle over control between her and the therapist. It could also be expected that she would pull for the therapist to direct the treatment, but then fight against this direction, representing her deep internal conflict. If this conflict manifested in the transference, there would be an opportunity to explore the feelings that this control dynamic evoked and to apply this knowledge to real-life situations.

COURSE OF TREATMENT

Therapy began with establishing a therapeutic alliance and Emily's setting initial goals of increasing independence in decision making, recognizing that certain aspects of her life were outside of her control, and adjusting to motherhood. What followed was an examination of her strategies to cope with stress and manage uncomfortable emotions, including her use of obsessional defenses, leading to an increased awareness of the changes she wanted to make in her life. As she became aware of the burden of this way of coping, and what was behind it, she became more aware of her complicated feelings of anger, dependency, and struggle with autonomy and guilt.

In the next phase of treatment she acknowledged and described these feelings much more clearly. We attained a deeper understanding of her family dynamics, particularly related to her relationship with her mother, and this facilitated an understanding of her guilt and anxiety as manifestations of her anger. Increased awareness, acceptance, and tolerance of anger allowed Emily to confront it, and subsequently modify her behaviors and relationships with the goal of becoming an independent and confident woman and increasing her focus on her marriage rather than her family of origin. In this third phase of treatment, Emily was able to develop new and more accurate perceptions of her parents, and develop new ways of being close with her daughter and husband.

During our early sessions, Emily smiled as she greeted me, and then began to tell me about her week before she could even get settled in her chair. She spoke eagerly and at length about her difficulties with following through on tasks and making decisions, readily providing a multitude of examples. With ease, she shared tales of her agony about choosing one seat at a family dinner over another, selecting the perfect outfit for her new daughter, or organizing a large event for her company, all while maintaining a pleasant tone and a slightly disconnected facial expression. She repeated herself in session, which I imagined was a display of her internal experience of her thoughts as an endless loop. She continually talked about the challenges that were created by the birth of her daughter, and the guilt caused by her perception of the baby as an obligation rather than a source of joy.

She overlooked that making decisions, completing tasks, and feeling confident were tough for her even before having a baby. She had phone calls and e-mails accumulating at work, many events hosted by friends and family that she felt compelled to attend, and a long list of overdue thank-you notes to write for baby gifts. She acknowledged the change from running her own regimented schedule to having it controlled by a baby, who needed frequent feeding, changing, and naps. Emily lamented the loss of the life she had had pre-baby, and matter-of-factly and unconvincingly (to me) stated that it will somehow get better. It was easy for me to maintain objectivity, as it seemed Emily even spoke about her burdens and obligations in a slightly detached way, as though they were someone else's. At the same time, I empathized with her feeling overwhelmed by her responsibilities and could relate to her desire to evade them.

In this first phase of treatment, she was seeking reassurance that she would adjust to motherhood in ways she believed came naturally to everyone else. Her ambivalence about therapy was readily apparent. She would often make comments about how it was difficult for her to take time away from work for therapy, but rationalized that it would not be such a burden since she anticipated that the course would be brief. She was also initially ambivalent about her connection to me, which was not revealed until later.

The only indication early on that she questioned whether I was someone who could relate to and help her was when she asked me if I was a mother, and showed a tinge of disappointment when I responded I was not. I was a little disheartened because I knew it was not the answer she hoped for and wondered whether this self-disclosure tested her faith in my ability to identify with her. She did not admit until much later her initial discomfort with seeing a therapist who was about her age (in part, because of advice she had received from friends), and, not surprisingly, her belief that an older, more maternal and seasoned therapist would be the best fit. When she finally revealed this, she also told me that she looked forward to our sessions, and how she felt at ease ("as though you are a friend") and not scrutinized. Although I knew her compliment was sincere, it also seemed that she was trying to avoid overtly insulting my qualifications through her praise for my "doing a good job." This seemed to be an example of defensively doing and undoing, as she tried to avoid any negative feelings about me. Although this is a defense that she would later need to acknowledge, in that moment she deserved praise for allowing herself the freedom to defy her friends' advice, suspend judgment, and form her own opinion.

Once the alliance was established, her transference toward me was strongly positive, and she frequently told me that she thought about therapy in between sessions and wondered what I would think of an interaction or incident she had during the week. She sometimes came into sessions smiling, saying that I will be proud of her for making a decision or doing something she had been avoiding because of anxiety.

Although we did not explore it much in the therapy, her transference was not to a friend, as she had stated, but rather to a loving maternal figure, representing some transfer of her dependency from her relationship with her mother to our relationship.

While I suspect this transference was drawn from her idealized view of her mother, I also looked for evidence of transference to an overbearing, controlling mother who tells her what to do. An obvious negative transference did not develop, though there was a slight alliance rupture when I recommended that Emily start a selective serotonin reuptake inhibitor medication for postpartum depression and anxiety. I had recommended medication early in treatment, but she was ambivalent and, despite feeling overwhelmed and experiencing symptoms of an anxious depression, was functioning reasonably well at work and at home. We mutually agreed to hold off on medication and reconsider if her symptoms persisted or worsened. However, as therapy progressed, she felt ever more certain of not wanting to take medication. Her choice was fixed, but her reasoning transformed over time, initially based on achieving change without the assistance of an external and artificial source thereby maintaining control, and later based on her association of medication with a certain severity of illness she did not believe she faced.

An early goal of therapy was empowering Emily to make decisions, attempt tasks that she had previously depended heavily on others to do, and to become more tolerant of situations that were out of her control, such as almost everything involving an infant! We started with understanding Emily's use of obsessional defenses (doing and undoing, reaction formation, isolation of affect, and intellectualization) to avoid dealing with her intense emotions and the effect of this internal conflict on her marriage and experience of motherhood. With this in mind, I encouraged her to discuss many examples from daily life of her compulsivity, indecisiveness, and reliance on her mother, and in doing so, she started to recognize what she was missing in her life. She readily talked about how she coped with stress by instituting rules and routines, which were soothing and familiar and enabled her to feel "in control." She noted how much time she spent doing things like methodically washing baby bottles and plucking her eyebrows in a particular way, and was mildly frustrated about the time these rituals took away from other things that "should" be more important to her, like mothering her baby and nurturing her relationship with her husband.

Because she was not motivated to change the ritualized behaviors that distracted her from her anger and anxiety, we focused instead on identifying the potential consequences of marginalizing her husband to protect her relationship with her mother. She described a pattern where her mother offered an opinion, then her husband took the extreme opposite stance in order to regain some power within their own dynamic, and how this left her feeling that a decision would inevitably disappoint someone close to her.

After examining this sequence repeatedly in session, she came to realize her tendency to support her mother's view, which rendered her husband weak, as she consistently valued her mother's feelings above his. We discussed how she was more comfortable with disappointing her husband than disappointing her mother, because she knew from their shared history that their relationship would bounce back from the insult. This pattern was so ingrained that she did not see the cost to her marriage of repeatedly disregarding and devaluing her husband. Further, she projected onto him her anger and negativity toward her mother, which allowed her to distance herself from these powerful emotions and not deal with them.

She justified her mother's over-involvement with her fear that she could miss something important if she ignored her mother's advice, and also compared her limited knowledge of child-rearing to her mother's vast personal experience, stating wryly, "She's just trying to help." Her mother commented on all matters regardless of magnitude concerning anything from a specific dress that Emily must buy for her baby to wear for a special occasion to whether her baby was starting to talk on time. Emily felt that once her mother posed a question about Emily's parenting, she couldn't shake it. It became a loop in her brain that she reinforced with preoccupation until she got so frustrated that she either succumbed to it (most often) or disobeyed it on principle.

She also wanted her mother to think highly of her and altered her behavior so as to be consistent with her mother's expectations. For example, she once got out of work early and instead of rushing home to be with the baby, she took a detour by the nail salon and got a pedicure, a luxury she had not had for a long time. She anticipated her mother's glare as she walked in the door with plastic wrap sticking out of her shoes betraying her secret, and concocted a lie that wouldn't blow her cover. She feared losing her mother's adoration, and wanted to identify with her mother who gave so much of herself for her children; however, it was important for Emily to acknowledge that that "selflessness" was her mother's way of indulging her own needs and that Emily needed to do so as well by carving out alone time, which would ultimately make her a healthier mother for her baby.

During this first phase of treatment, Emily and her husband traveled out of town for a friend's wedding and left their daughter in the care of Emily's parents. She was eager to spend some time with Evan, hoping it would resemble their pre-baby lives. While away, she found herself comparing their chemistry with that of other couples and was saddened by their lack of spontaneity and romance. She picked a fight with Evan, which had also become ritualized (with Emily telling him that he should have married someone more like himself and that their relationship was doomed, followed by her husband warning her that he may eventually concur if she reiterates it enough), and precluded the intimate tryst she had hoped for.

While discussing this argument, for the first time I sensed that Emily's behavior and reactions were ego-dystonic and that perhaps she was motivated for change. She was distraught over her inability to rein in her anger once it was triggered and that Evan received the brunt of it. She also hated how remorseful and guilty she felt in the aftermath. This enabled us to explore and understand her motivation for these outbursts, which was primarily to discharge her anger in an environment where it did not feel threatening and to seek reassurance from her husband. She did not fear that their relationship would be destroyed if she expressed anger toward him, as he came from a family where brutal honesty was common and she had enough history with him to know that their relationship would survive.

This conversation marked an important transition in therapy, and allowed us to shift toward a more careful observation and understanding of her parents in the next phase of treatment. For example, when she watched her parents interact with her daughter, she was struck by their level of intensity and focus, as they reacted to the baby's every move, fussed over her, and resisted going to the restroom unless the other one was intently watching her. It was confusing for Emily to watch because she perceived it as equally loving and overwhelming, with her mother intruding on the baby's space and her father singing silly songs and dancing around like a circus clown. She imagined that the effect on her daughter was the same (equal parts loving and overwhelming), and feared that her daughter would become inhibited and dependent as well. In exploring the anxiety she felt when watching her parents with the baby, I speculated that that was likely how they parented her when she was a baby, but perhaps even more intensely since she was their first. As we explored this, she realized that they parented this way because they were anxious, not because they were overwhelming, controlling, and demanding by nature. She was increasingly frustrated with her parents for restricting her in this way, but also realized that it did not compromise her loving feelings toward them. We discussed this in our sessions as one way in which she was separating, maturing, and becoming more attuned to reciprocity in relationships.

Once she was able to tolerate some frustration with her parents over their parenting style, she started to feel, accept, and tolerate anger in a way she had not experienced previously. We then focused on developing her ability to experience and tolerate ambivalent feelings toward others without feeling like her anger put her relationships in jeopardy. I figured that her parents' advice and involvement was fulfilling their own desire to be needed by her, but awaited further exploration before making this interpretation in session. If that was true and she accepted it, she could start letting go of her feelings of inadequacy and guilt over not being good enough, allowing her anger to dissipate and her confidence to grow.

As therapy progressed, she spoke of frequent situations in which she was being influenced by others, most notably her parents, but also her girlfriends and coworkers. As we discussed these interactions, she spoke louder and more emphatically, and I sensed true annoyance in her voice. I pointed this out to her and she agreed that all of the unsolicited advice and overpowering opinions infuriated her. I validated her anger, empathized with it, and accepted that it was a natural response to an oppressive situation. We then had an opportunity to explore the actual experience of feeling angry and why it was so anxiety-provoking that she needed to avoid it.

Her increasing awareness and acceptance of her angry feelings let her look more directly at her relationships within the family. She was particularly concerned that if she did not examine the "real" relationships she had with her family members and change her attitude and behavior, her daughter would be negatively affected by having a wishy-washy mother. Despite gaining this awareness and *wanting* to change this pattern, she ruminated about making decisions or taking initiative week after week without taking action. It was essential that I maintain an active stance and be persistent in encouraging Emily to practice (or even imagine practicing) a different approach than usual. Her natural inclination to not make waves seemed to win over every time.

After many weeks of discussing this pattern in therapy, Emily presented for a session and revealed that she had confronted her mother while they were out for a weekend brunch. She felt empowered to share her mounting frustration with her mother, and believed the gathering of people was appropriate for the conversation she wanted to have, as only the five members of her nuclear family were present. She thoughtfully and carefully told her mother that she appreciated her assistance but did not want her unsolicited input on everything, especially pertaining to mothering, because it hindered her ability to gain confidence in independent decision making. Although Emily said this gingerly, her mother was instantly offended, started crying, and made melodramatic statements daring Emily to try to manage without her help. As expected, Emily's father and brothers sat quietly and did not diffuse the tension; Emily wasn't sure how they felt about what she said, but knew they wouldn't express it, even if they covertly supported her.

When she returned home and recounted the event to her husband, he was proud of her for letting her mother see a glimpse of the effect her mother's continuous involvement had had on her. In session, after she relayed this incident to me, I anticipated that she would feel remorseful, but she did not. However, she hated feeling like a villain for causing such a striking reaction from her mother. She reported that her interactions with her mother reverted "back to normal" by the next day, but she was sure that her mother would catalog the event and sprinkle remarks about it into future conversations. I pointed out the value in what she did—that is, that it was the first time she had acknowledged that her dependence was problematic.

Although it was readily apparent that it would not be productive to have recurrent conversations like the one they had, the experience was eye-opening for Emily. I encouraged her to utilize her increased insight into the situation to help her understand her mother's motivation for providing constant support and how it undermined her. This gave me an opening to interpret the dynamic I considered earlier, that her parents were so caught up in her and her brothers' lives because it satisfied needs of their own. She agreed and acknowledged that their involvement did not only signify that she needed them, but possibly that they also needed her.

It also opened the door to exploring Emily's role in perpetuating this pattern and how she could modify her own response to create better boundaries between herself and others. She realized over time that she constantly sought guidance from her mother and reinforced her mother's central place in her life. In this context, we discussed frequently how Emily's parents were the primary baby sitters for her daughter (including 3 days per week instead of full-time daycare) and how Emily heeded their parenting advice over recommendations given by their daughter's pediatrician. She confided that it was heartbreaking when her daughter would reach for Emily's mother instead of her, which she knew occurred in part because of her mother's integral role in her daughter's life. Experiencing more frustration with her inability to make choices solely on what is best for her and her "new" family helped to make her behavior more ego-dystonic. She worried about the potential negative impact she would have on her growing daughter if she remained indecisive.

Her greater readiness to change her behavior was a major achievement of the therapy, and set the stage for the next phase of treatment, namely the challenge of making her primary relationship that with her husband rather than with her mother, and feeling like she could be the mother she wanted to be. To this end, she started taking initiative in caring for her daughter in situations that previously seemed too daunting. She took her daughter to birthday parties for her friends' children unaccompanied by her husband and was the sole caregiver for a weekend when her husband was away at a conference (despite her parents offer to stay with her for additional support). Though these ventures did not go seamlessly, she coped with the unpredictability and gained confidence in her parenting skills through practice. Interestingly, she modeled her parenting style on what she observed with her husband rather than her parents, and responded as best she could to what she believed her daughter needed from her in the moment.

Gaining some independence from her mother enabled her to refocus her priorities and make her marriage more central. The honesty and transparency in her communication with her husband strengthened their bond, and were the characteristics lacking in many of her other relationships. In therapy, I encouraged Emily to appreciate Evan for his relaxed and unassuming nature, and to recognize how little effort their love required. She realized that she was taking him for granted and cultivating her other more demanding relationships for fear of losing them. She realized how much she enjoyed the simplicity of their time together and valued it over the social events she would have otherwise felt pressure to attend. I provided support and encouragement throughout this process, as I was genuinely proud of her and impressed by her maturity and willingness to examine and change aspects of herself she found undesirable.

TERMINATION

After 1 year of psychotherapy, Emily and I faced termination that was imposed by my residency graduation and transition to another practice. Although our relationship was ending, it entailed a beginning as well, because Emily planned to transfer her care directly to another therapist. In actuality, it was not that simple. I gave Emily the option to transition with me to my post-residency practice, but she felt logistically it would not be possible because of the additional commuting time required. It was unclear whether she was resistant to this change because of the actual logistics (which involved a total of an extra 30 minutes round trip) or because of her perception of the situation as insurmountable. Emily vacillated on this decision for several months, and also wavered on whether to continue therapy altogether, and I saw glimpses of the same woman who had presented initially—a composed and headstrong woman, ambivalent about therapy and fearful of the implications of accepting that she was suffering. Her indecision and quest for reassurance that she would function optimally without further professional help were clear evidence of her ongoing difficulties with decision making and asserting independence and her awareness of the need to continue therapy.

We explored Emily's feelings about termination with the undercurrent of her internal conflict about separation. Termination became one of the topics weaved into sessions for the last few months, and although I knew that it was difficult for her to show me that she was upset about ending with me, I believed it when she said so. She often jokingly made comments like "I can't believe you're leaving me!" and lamented over having to start with someone new, but quickly distanced herself from the sadness by commenting on how it may be fruitful to get a new therapist's perspective on the issues with which she was struggling. I sensed some shielded anger toward the situation (or me, perhaps), despite it being her choice to switch therapists, and inquired about this. She admitted to frustration with the arbitrary end of therapy, but asserted her decision to switch therapists. Her ability to convey how she felt improved as our last session neared, and she expressed how much she would miss our time together, a sentiment I shared and warmly conveyed back to her. In hindsight, I wonder whether she also transferred her care to minimize her dependence on me, just as she fought against dependence on her mother. Her ambivalence about following me and her need to be appreciative were also a replay of her feelings toward her mother.

ASSESSMENT OF PROGRESS

Toward the end of treatment, Emily was notably eager and more determined to explore her internal conflicts. She had a genuine motivation to change, but also a need to be a good patient and please me with her efforts. She had a strong desire to feel successful in every realm of her life, including therapy. Thus, her increased motivation stemmed not only from her increased insight and wish to accomplish as much as she could before we needed to end, but also from her connectedness to me in our therapeutic relationship.

It was that connection based on her true self that was one of her most significant achievements in therapy. She allowed herself to reveal her insecurities and her fears of not being loved by her daughter, losing her relationship with her mother, and not having priorities that aligned with those of her closest friends and extended family. The shame and sadness that were prominent when she entered therapy had lifted, and she was more open to challenging herself in her everyday life in ways that she had been unable to do previously. She accepted that she may not want exactly the same things as her mother or her girlfriends, and that

that did not mean she was flawed. It still produced a lot of uneasiness when she deviated from what she perceived as others' expectations of her, but became somewhat more tolerant of this feeling and noticed how it passed when there weren't any dire consequences. As she started to focus more on her own needs and wants, she settled into a place where she could decline invitations without immense fear or guilt. She chose to spend time at home with Evan rather than try to appease everyone else, and as a result, appreciated their time together more and felt closer to him. It was certainly a work in progress as the end of our therapy neared, but significant first steps had been taken.

Emily's temperament, dynamics, and early relationships, incorporated with an already challenging period of life for many women, made her vulnerable to distress in the postpartum period, when she was forced to confront the realities of her indecisiveness and heavy reliance on others. Her enmeshment with her mother and obsessionality were not overtly problematic until she herself became a mother and felt unprepared for the changes that this role transition necessitated. She wanted so badly to shift naturally from being nurtured to being responsible for another life. Her self-doubt, anxiety, and sadness precipitated postpartum depression, which forced her to address the dynamics that she previously ignored.

The areas that she still needed to address were gaining greater emotional distance from her mother and reducing her compulsive behaviors. These therapeutic tasks were likely intermingled, as she utilized rituals to feel in control and to alleviate anxiety that was created by her incomplete separation from her family of origin. I was impressed by her ability to change as much as she had in the year that we worked together and am confident that with a longer course of therapy, she would make strides. With continued therapy, I imagine she would repeatedly test the waters by asserting herself as separate from her mother and then evaluate for repercussions, only proceeding after confirmation that their relationship was not threatened. After repeated advances in this manner, her anxiety would lessen, her confidence would build, and she would not second-guess, obsess, and scrupulously perfect every single thing she does.

In writing this chapter and reflecting on my experience with Emily in therapy, I empathized with her drive for perfection, her desire to achieve and maintain closeness in relationships, and her sincerity in wanting to be successful as a wife and mother. Throughout therapy and in my reflections, I related to the pressures on young women to thrive in many realms of their lives and to perceive motherhood as a blissful and effortless transition. The media and real-life examples of women who appear to make this role shift impeccably have reinforced this idea, with Emily's girlfriends and mother serving as key examples for her.

My identification with her not only facilitated empathy but also enabled me to be captivated by her personal anecdotes and grasp the underlying emotion even when the stories may have seemed monotonous. When I felt the emotion she was not overtly showing or describing, I could bring it to her attention, which helped move the therapy process along.

However, my identification with her may have also posed some difficulty. Like Emily, I felt that her anxiety was to a certain extent "normal" and that she was struggling in the same way as many other women trying to find balance in their lives. It was tricky to figure out how to normalize the situation while also addressing Emily's unhealthy defenses and excessive guilt. In hindsight (and after gaining experience treating many other women in the postpartum period), I wish I had put a greater emphasis on her pathological responses to stress earlier in the course of therapy, but realize that I may have been inhibited by my awareness that her current role transition was troublesome for many women and also not wanting to rupture our alliance.

In reviewing this course of therapy, I also wish I had addressed the transference more directly in our sessions. Especially because Emily had commented on feeling at ease with me "like a friend," it was difficult for me to acknowledge observations of her transference to me as a maternal or authority figure or delve into her experience of revealing her insecurities and candid emotions, which did not occur in most of her close relationships. It must have been uncomfortable for her to feel vulnerable in therapy, particularly when it was seemingly important for her to impress me with her accomplishments, and it would have likely been useful to explore this together and relate it to other aspects of her life.

I was fortunate to have gained her trust to facilitate this explorative journey in which her depression lifted and she started to become more self-aware and independent. I also learned a tremendous amount from her about how obsessional traits and behaviors that originate in a functional way may interfere with functioning in later stages of life, but can be modified through therapy.

CHAPTER 7

SERIAL KILLERS, MOVIE STARS, AND ERUPTIONS

A Case of Obsessionality

BRIAN A. SHARPLESS

Fred, a middle-aged man with obsessionality and a lifelong struggle with interpersonal closeness, was able to open up and develop a richer emotional life and new relationships through psychodynamic therapy. The therapist paid close attention to building a strong therapeutic alliance, introducing basic education about therapy, emotions, and the nature of choice, and carefully avoiding some of the traditional interpretive therapy techniques that could cause this patient to feel criticized or shamed. This careful, highly empathic stance required a lot of restraint on the part of the therapist, and allowed the patient to slowly become more comfortable. The approach seems to have paid off with significant therapeutic gains.

Some would suggest that this patient was not appropriate for psychodynamic therapy because of his rigidity and very limited support system. But, the chapter tells a different story—a man with much previous therapy who is able to make needed changes because he found a safe place to talk about himself and have a corrective emotional experience.

The patient's style of speech and behavior in sessions is somewhat idiosyncratic and became a valuable focus of discussion and emotional exploration when other ways to open up were more difficult. The case also illustrates the therapist's dilemma when a patient is making potentially dangerous decisions, and how a careful effort at understanding these actions can result in more adaptive perceptions and healthier choices.

The therapist's self-reflection about a prior relationship in his own family helped him understand some of his reactions to this patient and were helpfully discussed in supervision. He is candid about his assessment of the patient's progress and his curiosity about him after termination.

PRESENTATION AND CHIEF COMPLAINT

Fred was a 56-year-old Caucasian male. He was slightly over 6 feet tall and quite thin with a classically ectomorphic body type. His appearance resembled the filmmaker John Waters. His hair was darker than one would expect for a man his age, and almost always unkempt. Fred dressed casually and appropriately with one exception; he wore a watch that faced the opposite direction. When in session, he almost always sat with his legs crossed. However, when discussing distressing material he assumed a more unusual pose, with his crossed "over" leg curved back under his "under" leg in a pretzel fashion, with no apparent or expressed discomfort. He used his hands often when he spoke, and some of these movements appeared effeminate.

Fred's manner of speech was noteworthy. Though he was clearly articulate and of above-average intelligence (as indicated by both his level of theoretical abstraction and his vocabulary), he spoke in a rapid, pressured manner that was often circumstantial (viz., contained many irrelevant details) and sometimes tangential. A high baseline level of anxiety was apparent, and one could hear rapid and shallow inhalations of air as he briefly paused during narrations. His level of eye contact was fair. Fred was difficult to interrupt, and in the first few sessions I had the distinct impression that he would be content with no silence or interchange.

The content of Fred's speech frequently revolved around two topics in particular. He spoke often about the golden age of cinema and female movie icons (many of whom are no longer living), and was clearly captivated by the glamour and opulence of old Hollywood along with the over-the-top femininity of its starlets. The deeds of serial killers and mass murderers were the other primary draw of his attention, and his descriptions of their exploits conveyed a combination of surprise, fascination, and revulsion. When discussing either movie stars or murderers, his speech was fairly stereotyped, and he would repeat stories almost verbatim, replete with the same jokes and inflections, almost as if he were playing a recording.

Fred presented for treatment at a community mental health center where he saw three therapists prior to me. He was extremely detached from social relationships, and his 95-year-old mother was essentially his sole regular contact. He expressed strong resentment toward her, his sister, and women in general for the preferential treatment and easier navigation through life that he perceived they received. He quickly yet somewhat superficially disclosed confusion over his identity and strong feelings of guilt as a result of his sexual attraction to men. This guilt and confusion were coupled with the belief that he would be happier had he been born female. His difficulties with self-image, however, extended beyond his gender, and he described a consistently low self-image and self-dissatisfaction.

Emotions were problematic for him in general, though his insight into these difficulties *as* difficulties was quite limited. Overall, he struggled with expressing, tolerating, and naming emotional states. When such material surfaced, he experienced it as threatening, his voice would rise in volume, and he would then become quite agitated.

Fred also viewed the world as extremely threatening. He feared interpersonal contact, but seemed to be drawn to it as well, as he was an avid walker in public areas. However, he often experienced paranoid thoughts and mild referential delusions during these excursions. For instance, when walking by young people, he sometimes believed he heard slurs directed at him, such as "Hey, faggot!" When he would chance upon an actual interaction with a person, he experienced debilitating levels of anxiety mingled with self-reproach (and sometimes fear of bodily harm). Interestingly, Fred also reported that he occasionally and, from his standpoint, seemingly unexpectedly became involved in potentially dangerous situations. During these times, he reported being at risk for being hurt, sexually assaulted, or killed.

Fred also reported enormous difficulty taking action and a general lack of motivation. Even when faced with what most would perceive as low-pressure and low-consequence decisions, he became stultified by the myriad consequences and possibilities. This indecisiveness made managing day-to-day affairs difficult, and he sometimes met with a case manager for assistance. She reported that his house was quite cluttered, as Fred hoarded objects such as deodorant cans, newspapers, and old magazines.

The eventual death of his mother was also a matter of great concern to him. He feared the possibility of an existence in her absence, and lacked confidence in his ability to manage his life at a practical or emotional level. Overall, his stated goals for therapy were nebulous and vague.

HISTORY

Fred's history is interesting and enigmatic. As he is a fairly poor historian who experienced difficulties recalling certain dates (e.g., the death of his father when he was 41), I supplemented my early clinical interviews with medical record reviews. He was born to his married parents, Alan and Christine. Alan was a professor at a local college and Christine was a homemaker. He has one older sister (from whom he is estranged) and no brothers. No early physical difficulties were reported and Fred met appropriate developmental milestones on time. Fred reported that his early childhood was "happy," but described his upbringing as "overly strict" and "puritanical." His family traveled often during this time, and he fondly recalled long trips to Europe. Based on these narratives, these trips appeared to be the first time he began to feel alienated, and he would spend time alone on these trips whenever possible

One chart entry mentioned a homosexual experience at age 11. The writer of the report intimated that his parents knew of this event, but Fred never disclosed it during treatment. When prompted, Fred reported that something had happened, but he seemed unable to provide clear details.

Early adolescence was a very difficult time for Fred, as his alienation increased and his relationship with his parents deteriorated. Fred began feeling and acting more feminine at age 14. This manifested subtly at first, but other children noticed he was less "tough" and sports-oriented than his peers. Though he had no close friends, he recalled a number of acquaintances who were kind to him. At some point during 10th grade, Fred decided that he wanted to be a girl. His increasingly feminine behaviors (e.g., exaggerated hand movements and a slight lisp) did not exactly endear him to his early 1960s male classmates, and he was picked on mercilessly. He painfully recalled being called "squirrely Fred," a somewhat antiquated term for a person of questionable or "crazy" character. During this time he also began to envy and resent his sister because she was "privileged" (viz., had less responsibility plus more care and protection from others) by virtue of her being a female.

He described his mother as manipulative and controlling. Nothing ever pleased her and he felt like he always fell short of her lofty ideals of perfection (especially in terms of his burgeoning homosexual desires and gender confusion). She would often break down and cry to enlist his father's aid in dealing with Fred. Although Fred often described Alan as a passive figure, he recalled receiving severe tongue-lashings from him. However, he also felt a kinship with Alan (and some pity), who was also dominated by Christine.

Needless to say, his relationship with his parents was strained during this time. Feelings of guilt over his gender and sexuality became pronounced. He began to have difficulties managing his feelings and would tear pages out of books and throw objects out of anger. He was dumbfounded by the incongruities between the world as presented by his parents, and the world as it "actually was" in school (e.g., people drinking, having sex, lying, and engaging in other seemingly "sinful" behaviors). More generally, he was troubled by the discrepancy between what he was taught to do and feel and what he actually wanted to do and feel. He was simultaneously scared and intrigued by the differences.

These feelings of anger and resentment did not abate, however, and led to more desperate actions. At 16 or 17, he bought sleeping pills to overdose on and a razor to slit his wrists. Although he did not make an attempt on his life at the time, he reported a great deal of suicidal ideation. And in spite of his natural curiosity and intellectual gifts, he was unable to bring these to bear for school, and further retreated into fantasy and isolation. Many of these difficulties in adolescence continued and intensified with age.

Fred graduated from high school in the lowest 5% of his class. Following graduation, he matriculated to a university in the southwest. After one month of classes, however, his parents took him home. Soon after, he was hospitalized for an "inability to control his emotions." The following year, he returned to the inpatient unit for a 5-month stay. His treatment regimen at this time included both psychotropic medications and electro-convulsive therapy (40 separate treatments). When questioned about this particular stay, he said that he had no idea what prompted the hospitalization, but records indicated angry outbursts/tantrums at home. It is unclear whether this regimen was excessive or warranted by the extremity of his behaviors.

At age 23, and against the wishes of his parents, he decided to travel alone across the country and had several noteworthy experiences. In the Pacific Northwest he reported having a brief, but meaningful, romantic/sexual encounter with a man. He recalled this experience often in sessions, and viewed this man as a "special case" and exception to his generally negative view of others. This positive experience during his travels was greatly overshadowed by several frightening events, however. At some point during his time "on the road" he became suicidal, and his parents retrieved him again.

His life afterwards was fairly stable, yet constricted, and he returned briefly to school and workforce training. Fred reported no other significant events until age 31, a time period corresponding to his parents becoming increasingly exhausted with his care. Tensions erupted when Fred became angry and threw hot soup in his father's face. Alan reacted by stabbing Fred in the leg with a fork. This resulted in another hospitalization (his last), and upon discharge Fred was provided with county-funded housing, medications, and both group and individual therapy. He became disillusioned with medications, and refused them after several years. His use of therapy dwindled as well, and his situation remained fairly unchanged until Fred was 48.

At that time Fred moved to a different catchment area. This resulted in new living arrangements (he now lives in a larger apartment building with more people with mental health problems) and a request by him to recommence individual psychotherapy at the community mental health center. Records indicate that he continued to have no contacts besides his mother and occasional calls from his estranged sister. He spent his time walking around the city visiting bookstores and other shops, watching old movies and reading alone, and eating fast food. A year before Fred began to work with me, he was provided with a new case manager who was quite diligent and took an interest in his care. She became a good and stable force in his life, helped him manage his financial affairs, and provided additional order.

CORE PROBLEM AND FORMULATION
Part I: Summarizing Statement

At the time of intake Fred was a 56-year-old man on disability with a long history of multiple hospitalizations, social isolation, a limited ability to tolerate emotions, and gender and sexuality confusion. Though he yearned for greater connections, especially with men (which sometimes resulted in dangerous situations), his unusual mannerisms, preoccupations, and pervasive suspiciousness generally kept others at a distance. Fred's mother, his primary social contact, was described as a critical figure who never truly accepted him. His pervasive feelings of differentness, self-criticism, and shame intensified with puberty and the increasingly complex social demands of school and work. These feelings led to angry outbursts, suicidal ideation, and long periods of time spent in fantasy.

Part II: Description of Nondynamic Factors

Fred has carried a number of diagnoses over the past 40 years, including schizophrenia, several personality disorders, and bipolar disorder. Both parents were reported to suffer from anxiety and a maternal aunt appears to have experienced some form of psychotic disorder. When he presented at the community mental health center, he was diagnosed with schizoid personality disorder and obsessive–compulsive disorder (OCD) based on semistructured interviews and residual schizophrenia based on paperwork from the referring county agency. Upon transfer to me, additional assessment and record reviews took place. Of note, I found no evidence of schizophrenia beyond paranoia and referential thinking. Thus, I modified his primary descriptive diagnosis to schizotypal personality disorder in order to capture these symptoms as well as his limited social network and odd mannerisms. I also assigned obsessive–compulsive personality disorder (e.g., due to his perfectionism, excessive doubt, inability to take action, and moral rigidity), OCD (hoarding), and gender identity disorder.

Fred was likely a "high-strung" child who began to isolate himself and have peer difficulties in elementary school. He also appears to have experienced at least one sexual trauma in childhood (and several attempted sexual assaults as an adult). Social difficulties and emotional lability intensified with age, and he received electro-convulsive therapy and several bouts of medication during numerous psychiatric hospitalizations. He is currently averse to psychopharmacology due to the "personality changes" he fears will result.

Part III: Psychodynamic Explanation of Central Conflicts

Fred's core psychodynamic problem is obsessionality. His main conflicts revolve around themes of aggression and anger, guilt, autonomy, loss of control, and closeness (i.e., sexuality in the narrow and broader senses of the term). He also suffers from intense guilt associated with maternal expectations and wishes. With this core problem, the formulation was primarily situated within the ego psychology framework.

Fred's history indicated many early difficulties with experiencing and regulating affect. One could reasonably hypothesize that his nervousness and sensitivity were a poor fit for a critical and intrusive parent. His emotions were likely not properly contained and tolerated, and as a result they became imbued with the scary levels of intensity so characteristic of childhood experiences (i.e., strong feelings of fear, power, responsibility, and guilt). As an older child, he quickly incorporated, yet did not completely assimilate and digest, the family prohibitions of behavior. However, he realized that he could not live up to these ideals, and quickly felt resentment mixed with guilt as a result of so strongly disappointing his parents. He avoided these feelings through physical isolation, intellectualization, isolation of affect, and fantasy.

At times, however, his typical obsessive defenses broke down. One notable event occurred at age 21, in the wake of Fred having a brief romantic encounter with a man from a nearby city. When this came to the attention of his family, an argument ensued, and harsh words were exchanged. As the situation reached a fever pitch, Fred slapped his mother's face and angrily blamed her for his homosexuality. Immediately afterwards, he avoided being alone with her for fear that an explosion of anger would recur if she "pushed" him again. This avoidance became something of an act of contrition for this fearful expression of anger and resentment. He seemed to realize at this time (if not consciously), that there were frightening consequences to be had for both himself and his family if these suppressed/disavowed feelings of anger and resentment were given free rein.

Anger was not the only affect kept in check, however, and other "eruptions" of id impulses occurred. While on the solo trip across the country, he stayed at a YMCA in San Francisco. Against his better judgment and a "gut reaction" that "something was wrong," he visited the room of a particular (and peculiar) man who was also staying there. Fred reported that "something" drew him to this man. This person quickly became aggressive with Fred, however, and looked at him "with homicidal intent." This alarmed Fred greatly, and though he ultimately escaped the situation largely unharmed, Fred feared throughout this encounter that he would be beaten and sexually assaulted. In this instance, Fred's strong desire to be intimate with another man caused him to enter a life-threatening situation. His sexual and emotional longing superseded his concern for safety and self-preservation. As would be expected, his desire for connection almost always conflicted with internalized prohibitions against homosexual sex and, more generally, consorting with the "wrong types of people." In this case, however, the former (i.e., desire for connection) overwhelmed the latter, and with alarming consequences. The extremity of this situation and the way in which it validated his fundamental beliefs that people are dangerous and the world is unsafe (i.e., that his parents were right) caused him to return home and more generally limited his independence.

Since he began living alone, Fred was in fairly good control of his emotions, at least insofar as they are suppressed and do not often arise in unanticipated ways. He adopted a number of additional strategies to manage these feelings, and some of these include attempts to control others. Unfortunately, this way of being had a number of deleterious consequences for him. Most notably, he was unable to stay in touch with his feelings in relationships, and this left him often confused, and stultified in inaction when faced with even the most inconsequential of choices.

Similarly, his continuing preoccupation with film stars and serial killers served many psychological purposes, and was clearly in line with Waelder's (1936) "principle of multiple function." For instance, classic films for Fred provided an escape into an unreal world of fantasy where he was able to identify with beautiful and powerful women who easily attracted the attention of men (i.e., a wish). Films also allowed him to connect with his father, who was also a great lover of films, and who often took Fred to the cinema. Further, the films he gravitated toward were the films of his youth, prior to the painful derailments he experienced in later life, and when life seemed rife with possibilities.

His interest in serial and spree killers was similarly complex. After much exploration of Fred and his intrapsychic functions, it became apparent that his captivation with serial killers provided a sublimation and partial discharge of his aggressive impulses (i.e., partial identification with the killer). He was titillated by their depravity, nonchalance for human life, and ability to freely enact their dark urges upon others while he simultaneously maintained a sense of moral superiority over these clear violators of humanity and the existing social contracts. Although these interests were organizing for Fred in some ways, they also served to keep him distant from others, and his frank discussions of these topics would "turn people off" and make him appear odd or uncouth.

A typical Core Conflictual Relationship Theme (CCRT) for Fred would be a wish to be in control of his emotions and "unacceptable" urges (especially anger, aggression, and sex), a response that others impinge upon his rights and attempt to wrest control from him, and a response of self that he is anxious, fearful, and disoriented.

Fred had a number of strengths that were readily apparent and sometimes related to his difficulties. Most notably, his natural intelligence made his obsessive defenses feel more "justified," and provided him a greater ability to rationalize and intellectualize. It also made him an interesting person to talk to, and this was somewhat seductive at times, occasionally leading us off-topic. Another of Fred's strengths was kindness. He became visibly upset when the rights of others are trampled upon, and although some of this is due to an unconscious identification, he was also genuinely concerned about others' welfare. Finally, Fred displayed an ability to persevere in the face of adversity. Although profoundly fearful of others' intentions, he held on to the hope that things could get better, as indicated by his daily perambulations and seeking out help from therapists.

Fred appeared to have been temperamentally neurotic and suffered from nervousness, anxiety, and negative affect in general. There seemed to be a family history of this temperament as well. The combination of his sensitivity and reactivity likely made his inner life more intense, and therefore he became more vulnerable to fears of loss of control over his impulses. At these times, he attempted to return the situation to his control using many of the maneuvers described previously.

Further, speculatively, Fred's attraction toward men, and possibly his discomfort with his biological maleness, were likely innate, but his particular circumstances at home (especially, complicated relationships with the women in his family) interacted with and intensified these conflicts due to his perception of constant disapproval. Regardless of their ultimate origin, his homosexuality and gender identity dysphoria were both associated with a great deal of tumult within his nuclear family.

Fred's use of obsessive and schizotypal defenses served to maintain the status quo of both his symptoms in general and his interpersonal fears in particular. For instance, his attempts to maintain control over his emotions led him to place rigid boundaries on relationships with others. When individuals disclosed and invited reciprocal self-disclosure, Fred's feeling that he was losing control caused him to keep others at a distance and, in more extreme cases, actually alienated those who would otherwise be interested in becoming more intimate. In other situations his wishes for connection overloaded his defenses, led him to act out, and compromised his judgment. These events then served to reinforce his belief that the world, people, and intimacy were all fraught with danger (both emotional and physical), pain, confusion, and disappointment.

Part IV: Predicting Responses to the Therapeutic Situation

A realistic appraisal of Fred's prognosis needs to take into account the following: (1) the long history of his difficulties, (2) the long history of treatment without apparent change, (3) his increasing behavioral and interpersonal rigidity with age, (4) a paucity of interpersonal contacts, (5) ambivalence about changing his way of being in the world, and (6) the possibility that a recurrence of "eruptions" could severely derail treatment and potentially place Fred in physical or emotional danger. Thus, structural change was likely to be very slow, and it was unlikely that he would markedly change during the limited time (viz., 2 years) allotted to us. Further, any sort of hard-won change likely required a great deal of repetition, sensitivity, and attention to the therapeutic alliance. It was likely that Fred would take quite some time to move toward the middle phase of treatment, as the alliance and early interventions would progress at a gingerly pace.

From the first session it was apparent that the suspiciousness and fear of criticism that permeated Fred's overall life also infused our sessions. Thus, he would likely view me as a punitive, impinging other who may not have his best interests at heart or who may be "corrupt" or "immoral" (i.e., not the "right" therapist). His pervasive fears would also likely lead to difficulties in connecting with me and trusting me enough to disclose painful material. Typical therapeutic interventions (e.g., confrontations, interpretations) were likely to be experienced as my painfully controlling (and disorienting) him. Thus, therapy required a delicate balance to be both comfortable for him and "therapeutic."

He would likely adopt several unconscious strategies to keep emotions in check and anger at bay. Most notably, the rapidity and circumlocutions of his typical manner of speech would help ensure that he maintained control over both the content and the depth of his narratives. He would likely react to attempts to go "deeper" (via expressive interventions) as if they were ego impingements and unwanted penetrations. These feelings would likely lead to increased agitation and even fewer pauses. Functionally, his speech would provide an illusory (and ambivalent) sense of closeness between us which would be comforting, but also result in prohibitions against going further.

COURSE OF TREATMENT

Overall, the course of treatment was slow, yet steady, and at times it was punctuated by more dramatic events. As expected, the alliance was established neither quickly nor easily, and it remained fairly brittle for the first few months. Agreement on goals and tasks was hindered by suspiciousness, ubiquitous fears of negative evaluation if he were to disclose "shameful" things, and his pervasive tendency to control the content of the session via rapid-fire speech and quickly alternating topics. My familiarity with old movies and serial killers facilitated the bond component of the alliance, however, and allowed for initial forays into his history and emotional world. It served the dual purpose of being a safe way to "connect" with me without *really* connecting more meaningfully, and also provided a common language for discussing life matters with treatment salience. Striking a balance between the clear utility of these types of "familiar" discussions on the one hand, and not overly gratifying him or enabling his tendencies toward intellectualization on the other hand, proved to be quite challenging. I usually avoided these threats to treatment through not disclosing my personal tastes in films, and maintaining the focus of discussions on Fred, using my knowledge of films only to trigger and subsequently elaborate upon his emotional and interpersonal experiences.

Fred's manner of speech and the indirectness of his expressions of affect were impediments to therapy and they became prime foci early in treatment. His mode of speech could be overwhelming, and made me feel as though there was relatively little space for me in sessions. In response to this presentation, I began to incorporate several supportive and expressive therapy techniques. Along with reality testing and use of clarifications, I began to pay careful attention to his tone, rate of speech, and nonverbal communications. I began to notice shifts when they occurred, and then later (empathically) inquired into what may have prompted them (e.g., "I notice that your thoughts are really racing right now, and wonder if your feelings about the difficult experience you just told me about may be related to that"). In many cases, he was fairly oblivious to his behaviors (e.g., twisting his legs when agitated). By tentatively (and repeatedly) linking these manifest behaviors to the fact that feelings are what ultimately appear to give rise to them, we both began to develop a better understanding of his emotional world.

I asked permission to note the changes in speech and thinking when I saw them occurring "in the moment" as a precursor to our beginning to look at these matters more deeply. He agreed and this way of working together simultaneously respected his sensitivity toward feeling controlled and allowed me to intervene more directly. I also noted the pervasive criticality and inflexibility of his self-judgments. The combination of these interventions slowly reduced his circumstantiality and tangentiality in session and began to bring his pervasive self-criticism and self-judgment into conscious awareness.

Concurrent with this work on exploring shifts in affect was psychoeducation about emotions and the nature of choice and action. In all honesty, I should have focused much earlier on choices and action, but I was cautious because all the early attention I directed toward his emotions left him puzzled and annoyed. I explained that emotions can be important sources of information about what we want and do not want, and noted the limits of rational thought for making many of the important decisions in life. We also discussed relevant philosophers (especially the Danish philosopher Kierkegaard). Specifically, I proposed that most of the important decisions people make contain nonrational components (including unconscious wishes) that are no less important, and may actually be *more* important than rational ones. I proposed that this requires not only courage in the face of uncertainty, but also a commitment to a course of action. Though abstract and theoretical, these discussions chipped away at his defenses in a supportive, complimentary way and served as an important segue to his everyday difficulties with action. Action and inaction became a recurrent topic during our sessions, and we later incorporated the many "shoulds" that permeated his internal world (i.e., "You should be 'straight'", "You shouldn't get angry," "You should always be polite").

I often asked, "Where is that voice coming from?" when his demeanor shifted while articulating self-judgments. He soon recognized that he was indeed speaking with his mother's voice and not his own. Following this insight, the work of dampening overly harsh introjects and incorporating flexibility into a rigid system required a shift toward more expressive dynamic techniques. Although I used interpretations sparingly with Fred due to their potential to be too affectively laden and disorienting to him, I frequently used confrontations and "partial interpretations" (Glover, 1931; Rockland, 1989) to reduce the power of these introjects.

As one example of a partial interpretation following a disclosure of his homosexual desires, I noted:

"Thoughts like that must be very troubling to you, and also make you feel enormous amounts of guilt [*empathic reflection and mild intensification of existing affect*]. It seems to me that you've taken on at least some of these thoughts from the critical interactions you described with your mother [*a benign projection locating responsibility for the problem partly outside of himself*]. I also wonder if this is the only way that you can view them [*raising the possibility that other judgments and experiences are possible*]. From what I know about you, it makes sense that you would feel this way, but I imagine that it's still fairly uncomfortable [*empathic statement*]."

In these interventions, only conscious contents were linked, and as noted in Summers and Barber (2010), empathic comments preceded and concluded the more expressive statements. These interventions that I have called "empathy sandwiches," made it less likely for him to feel criticized.

Along with his attempts to control both me and the therapy, Fred also often wondered whether I thought less of him following self-disclosures, or if I even laughed at him after sessions. He often experienced me as a critical figure, and this was perhaps most directly brought to light one day when he stated that, "You look like a priest today." We explored these various fantasies, and when I questioned him about them, Fred was usually able to distance himself a bit and engage in reality-testing/exploration. At other times, though, his fears became more intense. In these cases, I did not interpret the transference directly, but defused the intensity of it empathically noting that similar experiences could be found in his interactions with others ("It seems to me that you're experiencing me very similarly to that cashier at McDonald's").

This initial maternal transference (characterized by experiences of criticism) eventually became more erotic, and this slowly came to my attention following a few separate events during the span of a month. First, Fred reported several dreams involving me in thinly disguised romantic encounters. Second, he became mildly preoccupied with my sexual orientation, and wondered aloud if I was straight or gay (while acknowledging that he knew I would not disclose this). Finally, after several sessions, he disclosed his attraction to me and his romantic fantasies about me. This disclosure was *immediately* followed by an intense barrage of self-flagellation, and critical judgments about his "disgusting behavior" and the absolute "inappropriateness" of having these feelings and sharing them.

The intensity of this self-criticism was jarring, and left me wondering how to optimally intervene. I decided that what would be most useful for him at that particular moment would be not to do too much confronting or interpreting. Instead, I empathized with how hard it must have been to share these feelings with me, and commented that this openness was a notable change from when we started working together. I also spent time trying to help him understand that such feelings in therapy are normal and reduce his powerful guilt through both noncritically tolerating and containing his emotions, and connecting his feelings to the therapeutic situation itself (i.e., the feeling of closeness that came from being listened to and understood by another man).

Although he experienced some difficulties returning to this topic, he became much less reticent discussing his sexuality. He also experienced less manifest guilt. In retrospect, this interchange over his sexual fantasies appears to have resulted in a corrective emotional experience (e.g., Sharpless & Barber 2012). That is, he reexperienced an old, unsettled conflict (i.e., acceptance of his homosexuality) with a new ending. This time, instead of being met with criticism and disgust, his wishes were met with acceptance and understanding.

With regard to countertransference, I experienced Fred as similar to a relative of mine with schizotypal traits. This person was an important figure in my childhood and adolescence, and I found myself wanting to help Fred as I would have liked to help out my relative (i.e., maximizing potentials and joy in life). I liked Fred's idiosyncrasies, and became very fond of him. I discussed my reactions with my supervisor, and we both surmised that this similarity/fondness explained some of my devotion to Fred. He noted that many therapists would have viewed Fred as a "supportive case" and seen little hope for change, but that I strove to push him more than others might have. However, my "closeness" to the case also led to some feelings of impatience at what I experienced to be a slow pace of progress.

Approximately 1 year into our sessions, I was able to see Fred the day after an "eruption" in which his desire for connection placed him at risk. Specifically, Fred had been walking around for several hours and found himself far from his apartment. It was late, and he was lost. This served as an opportunity for a man he had never met before to approach Fred and strike up a conversation. Soon after, the man offered him a ride home. Fred was very flattered by the attention and noted that the man looked "well-dressed, attractive, and normal enough," describing again how he bases his decisions on "superficial appearances" like attractiveness. Fred quickly agreed to the offer, but the situation soon turned dangerous. Fred noticed that they were not traveling in the appropriate direction. The man said that this was "fine" and that he wanted to go to his own house first and hoped Fred would not mind. As they continued driving, Fred expressed some trepidation about this change of plans. The man, by Fred's report, quickly changed demeanor, "like Dr. Jekyll into Mr. Hyde," and made his sexual intentions clearly known, expressing anger at Fred's hesitancy. Fred felt extremely frightened at this point and could not recall exactly how he convinced the man to pull over and let him out of the car.

In session, he presented this event in the same rapid-fire, tangential, and agitated manner that he had at the beginning of treatment. After clarification of the narrative, I said that "this sounds like a terrifying experience for you, and similar to other ones you've described. I wonder if it might be useful to understand how this situation arose, and to look at it in the context of other stories you've told me?" He agreed to this plan, and for the remainder of this session (and the next few sessions), we explored the moment-to-moment unfolding of both this event and his internal experiences.

Fred realized that he had been feeling lonelier than usual in preceding days. He felt like "a rat in a cage." He also disclosed that he had not seen a particular well-groomed man downtown in quite some time. Although he never spoke to him, Fred regularly saw the man at a local shop and was attracted to him and his absence troubled and preoccupied him. Fred also had an upsetting interaction with his mother over a prior holiday weekend. His sister "chose not to grace us with her presence," and his mother became very critical and attacked his sexual past during dinner. Viewing this congeries of factors together, Fred came to realize that his frantic desire and hope for any type of connection with the man in the car caused him to overlook numerous "warning signs" of malevolent intent.

Toward the end of treatment, Fred reported a more positive experience with a man named Jeremy who lived in his building. This relationship evolved rather slowly through chatting with each other in passing, and eventually Jeremy invited Fred out to a hookah bar. Fred was very excited yet disoriented by this, and the offer provided opportunities for me to view his conflicts and ambivalence around interpersonal situations and making decisions *in vivo*. He noted how Jeremy teased him and was hurtful when he criticized Fred for asking questions that he had just answered. He did not like these interpersonal barbs, but wanted to be near Jeremy in spite of the pain that it caused him. We explored the ambivalence in session, and he eventually decided to accept the invitation. However, the event also served to arouse paranoid fantasies, as Fred feared for his safety after dark, and worried that his mother would find out he was cavorting with a "not perfect person" who had some unsavory qualities.

Needless to say, the presence of another person in Fred's life besides his mother and me was quite a shift, and led to a great deal of in-session discussion about his conflicts around closeness. Although this first outing with Jeremy was not reported to have gone well (Fred's anxiety crippled his ability to make conversation), they soon became regular events. Not long after, Fred also began spending time socializing with another man. In spite of the fact that these were not "perfect people" who would be unfailingly kind and understanding to him, Fred maintained these connections throughout the remainder of our sessions. They served important, yet limited, supportive functions for him. I liberally used confrontations in order to encourage Fred to clarify what he actually wanted and what he felt during these social interactions instead of what he *should* want and feel. I also supported him by noting the courage it took to face his many fears and engage with others. Certain cognitive-behavioral techniques were employed during this time as well such as challenging rigid automatic thoughts and making predictions prior to entering feared situations and then evaluating the actual outcomes.

TERMINATION

As I was seeing Fred during my clinical training, we both knew there was a predetermined endpoint. Although I had hoped that working through my leaving would be useful for Fred, discussing it in a sustained fashion proved quite difficult. He had little manifest interest in examining this topic, and I had to become direct in my prompts (e.g., "I can't help but notice that we will soon be ending our time together, but that we haven't discussed this or any of your reactions to it"). Had I not directed him, I think he would not have broached the topic at all.

After easing into the issue in a more intellectualized, practical fashion by discussing who would be taking over his care and reviewing progress, we were eventually able to discuss some of his feelings about my leaving. While our last session was not as affectively loaded as others I have experienced, it did have warmth to it. He wished me well and asked about my next steps. Although I cannot recall his precise wording, he subtly acknowledged his recognition of the interest I took in his life, thanked me for my time, and noted that he would miss talking with me and had enjoyed our conversations.

ASSESSMENT OF PROGRESS

At termination, I was keenly aware that Fred still suffered considerably, remained isolated, and had limited joy and passion in life. However, substantive progress was made in at least six areas. First, Fred made gains in his ability to communicate and interpersonal functioning. Namely, his circumstantial and tangential speech decreased, and he was better able to discuss topics other than his two favorites. When more anxious, however, he regressed to the familiarity of his old speech patterns, but was better able to recognize this as a sign that he was upset about something. These changes and an improved ability to tolerate interpersonal fears allowed him to secure two platonic friends. Although strong ambivalence toward these relationships remained and he wondered if they were "the right people," they became a part of his life.

Second, his range of behavior became broader and bolder. Although his default narrative remained a paranoid one, it softened somewhat. Over time I heard less referentiality in his narratives, and this suspiciousness became more "general" (i.e., "They might have been talking about me" as opposed to, "They called me a fag").

Third, Fred experienced a reduction in the power of his negative introjects and subsequent guilt. Regarding the former, he readily identified introjects as introjects, and could better evaluate whether these were his own admonitions or the echoes of others. That is, his overly harsh superego softened. Following our discussions of his erotic transference and accepting my acceptance of these feelings, he could more easily own his other sexual wishes without extreme self-castigation. He was not as responsive to the introjected mother's critical view. Though much shame and guilt remained, his tolerance of these deeply human issues increased.

Fourth, Fred's healthy access to his emotions improved. He continued to fear the negative consequences of his feelings, but was able to recognize and apply emotional experiences to his life and allow them to help guide his actions. However, when under stress, all possibilities still felt apocalyptic in their intensity and he regressed to obsessiveness. Generally, reports from Fred and his case manager indicated that he made decisions more quickly and with less difficulty. He also achieved more emotional insight into his risky behaviors (eruptions). No further instances were reported during the remainder of our time together.

Fifth, Fred became better prepared for the eventual death of his mother. Though not described above, we examined this topic at length during many sessions, and Fred demonstrated strong tendencies to avoid the subject using his characteristic *modus operandi*. Per the report of his subsequent therapist, his mother passed away several months after our termination. Though clearly a significant loss to Fred (as it removed a strong source of support and stability), he was reported to have weathered the loss well.

Finally, Fred began to engage in more pleasurable activities and developed two new hobbies: bingo and painting. Painting was much more provocative and therapeutically relevant. Fred painted as a child and always wanted to return to it, but was very hesitant. After discussions of his reluctance and some encouragement from me, he made an initial attempt. This resulted in a great deal of self-criticism, and he ultimately tore up the canvas in frustration. Clearly, his perfectionistic tendencies also manifested in this context, as he noted extreme disappointment that he was not a better artist, "like van Gogh." After several months of discussions, reality-testing, and continued wondering by the therapist about whether the process or the outcome was what he was ultimately interested in achieving, he began to keep some of his paintings intact.

CODA

At the end of my time with Fred, I was left with a general feeling of "unfinishedness." I wished that I could have continued seeing him and helped him to amplify the changes listed above. I also found myself occasionally wondering about him, and hoped that he had not experienced significant setbacks or drifted further into fantasy and isolation. In all honesty, part of my motivation for choosing him as the subject of this chapter was to, in a sense, "check in" with him and see how he was. I needed to get his consent to use his case for this book; I had to contact him. When I called, he was surprised to hear from me, but clearly pleased. After presenting the purpose of the call, we chatted briefly and discussed the implications of being the subject of a case study. He was flattered, but hesitant, and I encouraged him to think about it and mail in the permission form if he agreed, but emphasized that there would be no repercussions for me or him either way. I reiterated this again at the end of our call. Overall, it was a very pleasant interchange. It also allayed some of my fears that he may be too paranoid at the prospect of exposing himself (even in disguised form) to the world to agree. Within a week, I received his signed consent form in my mailbox. I experienced this as a concrete expression of his trust in me and acknowledgment of our work together.

REFERENCES

Glover, E. (1931). The therapeutic effect of inexact interpretation: A contribution to the theory of suggestion. *International Journal of Psychoanalysis, 12,* 397–411.
Rockland, L. (1989). *Supportive therapy: A psychodynamic approach.* New York: Basic Books.

Sharpless, B. A., & Barber, J. P. (2012). Corrective emotional experiences from a psychodynamic perspective. In L. G. Castonguay & C. E. Hill (Eds.), *Transformation in psychotherapy: Corrective experiences across cognitive behavioral, humanistic, and psychodynamic approaches* (pp. 31–49). Washington, DC: American Psychological Association.

Summers R. F., & Barber, J. P. (2010). *Psychodynamic therapy: A guide to evidence-based practice.* New York: Guilford Press.

Wäelder, R. (1936). The principle of multiple function: Observations on overdetermination. *Psychoanalytic Quarterly, 5,* 45–62.

CHAPTER 8

SKATING IN CIRCLES
A Case of Fear of Abandonment

DANA A. SATIR
PATRICIA HARNEY
KIMBERLYN LEARY

The case of Jennifer, a self-described wanderer who runs from relationships before she can be hurt, is about a patient who experiences overwhelming feelings of loss and abandonment that lead her to engage primitive defenses. The therapist is remarkably honest and direct in describing her own emotions, uncertainties, and dilemmas as she helps the patient tolerate and come to terms with these powerful affects. The intensity and range of the interaction between patient and therapist is described in intimate detail and helps the reader understand the minute-to-minute choices the therapist made in working with this patient.

The case history describes the patient's relationship conflicts as they manifested in her personal life as well as the transference, and illustrates how progress toward greater trust in others (e.g., object constancy), can be made in a relatively short period of time. The therapist's attempt to help the patient live with her painful emotions and her struggle with how much to guide and direct the patient, speak to the struggles all therapists share with a patient like this. Authenticity on the therapist's part, and developing trust on the patient's part, were critical ingredients in the development of greater self-esteem and independent functioning in the patient. Finally, the therapist's uncertainty and curiosity about the patient after the treatment is over captures a feeling well known to therapists who connect deeply with their patients.

In this chapter, we describe the psychotherapeutic treatment of a 37-year-old partnered woman, Jennifer, whose core psychodynamic problem we conceptualize as fear of abandonment. Jennifer presented for psychotherapy on the advice of her primary care physician for the treatment of anxiety. Upon evaluation, her therapist (DAS) noted Jennifer's persistent feelings of being unwanted, her chronic experiences of loneliness, and her self-loathing. In her early adulthood, Jennifer maintained a nomadic lifestyle as a singer in alternative rock bands, seeking romantic relationships with men that promised financial and emotional security. At treatment onset, Jennifer had been living in the region for about 1 year, the longest time she had lived anywhere in many years. Several months before seeking treatment, she had begun a romantic relationship with a man with whom she hoped to experience a more mature, mutually gratifying partnership. However, she was plagued with fears of his perceived infidelity. This chapter describes Jennifer's difficulties and the course of her treatment in which positive, though partial, gains are made over 8 months of twice-weekly psychotherapy. We explore the treatment relationship in detail as it relates to the conceptualization of her core psychodynamic problem. We also describe Jennifer's strengths, manifested in her curiosity, intellect, and resilience.

CHIEF COMPLAINT AND PRESENTATION

Jennifer contacted a community hospital for outpatient psychotherapy on the advice of her primary care physician for the treatment of anxiety after recently moving into an apartment with her current partner of 3 months. She arrived 30 minutes early for her first appointment. She was thin and tall, dressed casually in jeans and a loose fitting T-shirt, and was somewhat nondescript in appearance except for a frameless pair of eye glasses she wore, which created the appearance of a studious, much older woman.

I initially experienced Jennifer as friendly, pleasant, and intellectual. She had had several brief experiences with psychotherapy in the past, and described an interest in literature and the healing arts (i.e., meditation). She seemed comfortable talking about herself and presented a coherent narrative about recent events that led her to seek additional support. I was pleased I had been assigned to work with her. Jennifer seemed like an excellent candidate for twice weekly, psychodynamic psychotherapy. She had a curiosity about herself and her experiences, and possessed the capacity for self-reflection. I also remember feeling like Jennifer was trying to take care of me during Session 1—telling me repeatedly how much she enjoyed talking to me and looked forward to meeting me again. I felt the same sentiments (albeit with less intensity) listening to her and looked forward to our next encounter.

Jennifer described her concerns as more than anxiety; rather, she had a paralyzing fear that her current romantic partner (Ben) might leave or cheat on her. She stated that she was "obsessed" with the idea that Ben was with another woman, if, for example, he was late returning home from work and did not immediately call. Jennifer experienced her thoughts as intrusive and her worry as difficult to control. Since moving in with Ben 1 month prior to this presentation, she had repeatedly asked him about his loyalty and fidelity. When she was troubled by her anxiety around his whereabouts she would seek Ben's reassurance—did he love her? Was he intimately involved with another woman? Was he planning to leave her? Jennifer reported that Ben was "very understanding" and offered her support during these moments of distress, yet she feared if she continued these behaviors he may, in fact, leave because of her mistrust. She felt guilty that she questioned her partner when he had not given her any indication that he was unfaithful.

Jennifer also reported transitory, paranoid, or psychotic-like thoughts that accompanied these worries regarding Ben's fidelity. Occasionally, when feeling quite anxious, Jennifer heard messages from television, radio, or other people that she believed supported or challenged her fears. She helped me understand this experience during our session when I asked, "What is that like [the anxiety] for you?" She said that if people asked her questions during moments of heightened anxiety, she would take the phrases or words people used as validation that her fears were founded. In other words, she wondered why I would ask her about her anxiety, unless she had a reason to be anxious (i.e., my partner is cheating on me)? Jennifer also fixated on words or phrases from media that might offer "clues" to the anxiety she was experiencing or details around Ben's alleged affairs. Jennifer acknowledged that on some level she knew these beliefs might not be true, but she also reported that she could not disprove the connections she was making in these moments of high anxiety.

Prior to moving in with Ben, Jennifer had been living in her parents' home in a small suburban community. She was employed by a local landscaping company and worked part-time. She had spent the majority of her adult life as a performer, singing and playing drums in the local music scene. To support her artistic lifestyle, she often worked as an administrative assistant but reported that she had never maintained a job for longer than 4 months because of her tendency to "wander." Jennifer had toured and lived in several different U.S. cities. She had returned to her hometown to "regroup" in the wake of her romantic and financial difficulties. Jennifer's parents had been willing to let her live at home, and she had been gradually saving up money and "getting things together."

Jennifer reported her life, outside of her worries, was mostly positive. She enjoyed "simple pleasures" such as reading literature in local
coffee houses, watching foreign cinema, and riding her skateboard
around town. She found her mood was bright and she experienced
less anxiety when she exercised regularly, meditated daily, and stayed
socially connected. Jennifer had the ability to experience calm and relaxation for extended moments but since moving in with her partner these
coping skills were no longer effective with the intense vulnerability and
anxiety she was experiencing. She felt the relationship "had to work"
because she "could not move back home," and this self-imposed pressure
increased her anxiety. She also feared that as her partner got to know her
better he would see things he did not like about her and that ultimately
she would be more exposed living with him. Her goals for treatment
were to first feel better and then understand why she felt such extreme
anxiety and suspicion when she logically knew this was not accurate.

HISTORY

Jennifer grew up in an intact family with an older sister of 3 years (Aly-
son) in a suburban area. She reported that her father and mother had
both worked full-time during her childhood but that they had financial problems. She recalled that her home was sparsely decorated and
that her house looked "weather-beaten" and was "the smallest" in their
middle-class neighborhood.

Jennifer had a history of addiction and recent sobriety from opiates. In eighth grade, she experimented with illicit substances (mostly
psychedelics). She reported that she often abused substances when she
was playing music at concerts and had taken them intermittently over
the past 20 years. She stated with some sense of pride that she never
actively "sought out" recreational drugs, but when others offered them
to her she rarely refused. Jennifer described her interest in using psychedelics as seeking "transcendence." She had stopped using psychedelics
several years before our meeting. When asked what led her to stop, she
reported that a friend had died of an overdose. His death scared her and
she "abruptly stopped."

Jennifer started abusing opiates around the same time she began
experimenting with psychedelics. Jennifer believed she developed a
"more serious problem" with opiates in her mid-twenties, a time when
she felt the drive to get intoxicated was "completely out of control." She
reported that over a period of 5 years she was often high several nights
a week. She was fired from several jobs because she repeatedly called
in sick after waking up hung over. Getting high also caused significant

difficulties in her romantic relationships. Once while in an intoxicated state, she attempted to harm her then boyfriend when she found him with another woman.

Jennifer had difficulty describing her past or present affective states. She denied discrete episodes of depression, but described long periods of "low mood." She called the absence of low mood "happiness." She reported one quasi-suicide attempt years before I met her, which occurred in the context of a breakup with a boyfriend. Her boyfriend's abandonment triggered an "awful state" of feeling from which she felt compelled to escape. At that time she cut herself on her arm but did not require or seek medical attention. She denied any other suicide attempts or self-mutilation, or a history of trauma.

Jennifer has a family psychiatric history for mood disorder and substance use. She reported that her father was an alcoholic and drank every night, often to the point of intoxication. She reported that her father struggled with irritability and explosive anger. Jennifer also reported a family history of paranoia, and possible psychosis, in her paternal grandmother.

When asked for an early memory, Jennifer recalled being 11 years old and dreaming of purchasing a skateboard she saw at a local store. She started a money jar to save up her allowance and babysitting money. After collecting pocket change and small bills for months, Jennifer hoped she might be able to buy the skateboard she dreamed of. She had just been playing outside and her mother had repeatedly called her to come down for dinner. She watched some of the neighborhood children play in the street outside from her second-story bedroom window when her parents presented themselves at the doorframe. They noticed the jar of money on her dresser and asked her what it was for. Excitedly, Jennifer explained that she too soon would have a skateboard like the other kids in the neighborhood. She recalled her parents erupted with laughter and told her she would never be able to buy it. It was a silly idea to think she could ever save up enough money to buy a skateboard that cost $200. Jennifer remembered staring at the walls in her room and decided at that moment that she never really wanted the skateboard in the first place. She also recalled committing herself to "never wanting anything again."

Jennifer said that both of her parents drank alcohol after dinner and her father drank significantly more than her mother. She and her sister often witnessed her parents laughing when they were drinking in the living area and it was one of the few times they appeared "connected" as a married couple. She remembered that her father would raise his voice at her mother for not "keeping the kids out of the way" when he was intoxicated. It seemed to Jennifer that her father, in particular, had not wanted to have children.

Jennifer had friends in the neighborhood while growing up, but she was "on the outside" of social groups and never had "real friends." She was an average to below average student despite her intelligence and she rarely studied. Jennifer remained close to two high school friends whom she could tell "everything" and who were "always there" for her.

Jennifer discovered her interest in music during middle school when she was at a neighbor's house and played with her friend's drum set. She enjoyed the rhythm of percussion and the way she felt transported to another place and state of feeling. She liked the experience of being completely transfixed by what she was doing. She played in a band with other neighborhood kids and "worshipped" Led Zepplin.

Jennifer had several long-term romantic relationships that she described as "co-dependent." She initially maintained a sense of aloofness in romantic relationships and felt drawn to men who would take care of her financially and emotionally. Jennifer reported that she never left her partners, but when they left her she made every effort to reestablish their relationship. She frequently used sex to seduce her partners, and there were repeated breakups with the same partner until the relationship was completely dissolved. These endings were often dramatic, associated with infidelity, betrayal, and verbally abusive behaviors. But when the relationship did end, a switch flipped. Jennifer would suddenly not want anything to do with the previous partner and would immediately look toward a new relationship.

Jennifer graduated from high school and attended one semester of community college. Since she had been a teenager, she had been unable to maintain stable employment for over a year, and reported that she was either terminated from jobs for inconsistent attendance or she would quit. Jennifer wished she could achieve financial stability. During some sessions she would become despondent about her perceived lack of professional and personal success. Prior to moving to the city, she had maintained jobs as both a landscaper and hair stylist for several months. When I met her, she seemed to be functioning at a more stable level than at any other period in her life and was earnest about her desires for change.

CORE PSYCHODYNAMIC PROBLEM AND FORMULATION
Part I: Summarizing Statement

Jennifer is a 37-year-old woman presenting to psychotherapy with significant anxiety about her current romantic partner's fidelity. She moved out of her parents' home and started cohabiting with her partner. This move was the catalyst for intensifying feelings of abandonment. She struggles with maintaining relational stability in adulthood, especially with romantic partners. When threatened with the end of a romantic partnership she becomes overwhelmed and engages in impulsive, often-times destructive behaviors. Jennifer has been a wanderer for most of her life—untethered to jobs or geography—and struggles with feelings of inadequacy and failure. She abused substances throughout adolescence and adulthood while touring as a musician and abruptly stopped using within the past 5 years. She has a family history of substance abuse, mood, anxiety, and possibly thought disorder.

Part II: Description of Nondynamic Factors

Jennifer meets criteria for anxiety disorder, not otherwise specified, and dysthymia. In moments of heightened anxiety, Jennifer also assumes random events are specifically designed to communicate things to her (e.g., when she feels panicky and is watching a TV program, she believes the content contains a message for her about her worries). While Jennifer's history of substance abuse makes her mood disorder history difficult to diagnose, she currently struggles with chronic low mood, hopelessness, and deficits in self-esteem. Jennifer's parents frequently abused alcohol during her childhood. Jennifer did not identify discrete past traumas but was severely emotionally neglected in her family system. She has not engaged in a regular psychotherapy, but does find some relief from her anxieties in the individual practice of meditation. She has never tried psychotropic medications for her mood or anxiety.

Part III: Psychodynamic Explanation of Central Conflicts

Jennifer's core psychodynamic problem is fear of abandonment. Her key conflicts include the wish for closeness and intimacy with fears of being unwanted and rejected, chronic feelings of loneliness, and persistent experiences of self-loathing. When all else fails, she deals with her fears of abandonment by leaving others. In this way, she does not experience the intense pain of rejection, and she may be able to convince herself that she did not want to be with or care about the other person because she is not the one left behind. She also is not forced to tolerate the uncertainty of wondering if/when someone may leave her by foreclosing the relationship. Jennifer's childhood was characterized by emotional and relational deprivation and she often felt unsafe.

These conflicts are evident in several aspects of her history. In the vignette about her saving for a skateboard, her parents mocked and shamed her efforts. Quickly, she rejected and denied these longings, pretending she no longer had these desires. From this moment onward she tried to master her ability to want/reject things decisively and quickly. These conflicts are evident in her struggles with romantic relationships.

On one occasion Jennifer attempted to harm herself after the end of a romantic relationship. She was trying distract herself from the emotional pain of loneliness and abandonment by creating tangible, physical pain that she could do something about and treat. Her desire for love and acceptance intensify significantly when she is engaged in romantic partnerships. Even when Jennifer's dramatic attempts to cope with her feelings of loss are acknowledged by her partners, she sees her attempts as futile (i.e., she is unable to prevent their leaving), and feels powerless especially when there is tension and dissatisfaction in the relationship.

Faced with repeated rejections and plagued by fears of abandonment, Jennifer has relied on the defenses of splitting, projection, and projective identification. Projection has been most distressing for Jennifer in her current romantic relationship, as she has repeatedly projected her fears of abandonment onto Ben. As she had made efforts to create a more enduring, mature relationship and decided to live with Ben, Jennifer's unmet childhood longings for unconditional care, love, and mutual connection have resurfaced. She is justifiably concerned that her behaviors will cause Ben to reject her, further confirming her own badness and exacerbating her longings for intimacy and closeness. Yet, she feels helpless and is easily overcome by her fears.

Jennifer is unable to resolve the conflict between her desire for connection and her deep fears of abandonment and rejection. She wants to become more of an "adult" and has made efforts toward higher levels of functioning. But her efforts have proven more difficult than she could have imagined and she struggles with feeling "homeless." In her abstinence from substances she is unable to numb or dull her feelings, and as a result is overwhelmed by the intensity of her affective experiences. She is ill prepared to cope with the great uncertainty that characterizes this stage of adulthood. For the first time, she is truly confronting her fears of being unlovable, as well as her grief about the neglect she experienced growing up and how her life trajectory might have been different if she had a foundation of love and support.

Jennifer's gifts of curiosity and intelligence will be great assets in her psychotherapy. Her micropsychotic episodes of delusional thinking during affective flooding suggest that her strengths may be compromised at times by the nature and intensity of her fears.

Part IV: Predicting Responses to the Therapeutic Situation

Jennifer is likely to use the defenses of splitting and projection with this therapist to contain her affect as the relationship deepens. These defensive efforts will likely intensify as termination approaches, and the core conflict of abandonment is reactivated.

Jennifer has decided to pursue psychotherapy at this time, and is committed to taking greater responsibility for her actions and how they affect others around her. She has never had treatment for her mood or anxiety, either psychotherapy or psychopharmacology. Given her family predisposition toward psychopathology, she is likely to benefit from a psychopharmacology evaluation. Jennifer may also have an attentional disorder and might benefit from more formal psychological testing, both attentional and otherwise, to determine the nature of her difficulties and possible contributions.

COURSE OF TREATMENT

I knew when the treatment started that termination might be one of the most important phases of therapy. Jennifer had come to a training clinic for her therapy partly because she did not have health insurance. My training would end 8 months after Jennifer and I started, and she was told about this early on in treatment. I was keenly aware of the rupture my ending therapy would likely create and how my departure would potentially activate her core conflicts. My supervisor and I agreed that the pacing of treatment would be important and that I would need to pay attention closely and early to Jennifer's potential attempts to "abandon" treatment or recruit me to end treatment.

I have chosen to divide the description of the treatment into three parts. In the first 3 to 4 months, Jennifer decompensated associated with the distress of her increased fear of abandonment. Jennifer's subsequent attempt to reject me, her primitive defensive maneuvers, and my strong countertransference response constituted the second phase. The last phase, lasting 2 months, was the termination of treatment.

In the first phase, Jennifer was very open and readily discussed her beliefs that the TV was communicating messages to her along with other aspects of her paranoid thinking. Even though these symptoms seemed discrete in nature, associated with extreme affective flooding, and unaccompanied by other difficulties with thought organization or reality testing, I worried about what else I would come to learn about her.

I was also concerned about her recent sobriety in light of all the new stressors she was experiencing, and whether her engagement in treatment as well as her new living arrangements would threaten her sobriety. Jennifer denied her concerns about relapse, and in fact, she was surprised when I suggested she was early in her recovery and sobriety.

She had attended a few 12-step meetings in the past but had found them "unhelpful" and "hokey."

Early on, I noticed that I felt a lot of worry about Jennifer. She, however, seemed much less worried about herself than I was. I was fearful about her unstable finances and her cavalier manner of self-care. For instance, she did not know how she would pay for her rent and yet she bought an iPod. She brought it to our sessions and told me how excited she was about it and what a good purchase it was. Was I being overprotective and maternal in my concerns, or was she being irresponsible and reckless? This would be the first of many occasions where I would experience Jennifer's use of projective identification—her disavowal of affects and transmitting to me unwanted and unprocessed feelings. I wondered if this was how some of Jennifer's partners felt when they were in the position of taking care of her—wholly responsible for her survival emotionally, financially, and otherwise. It was an awesome responsibility. I was afraid if I did not respond to more benign examples of her own neglect she might make more extreme efforts to get my attention or caretaking.

During the first month of therapy Jennifer and I found a comfortable rhythm. She had taken some positive steps early in her move and managed to identify two part-time jobs that pleased her (assistant yoga instructor and stocker in a food co-op). She began to earn more each week than she had ever before. While these were positive, early gains, most often Jennifer came to sessions discouraged and disappointed that she continued to repeatedly question her partner's fidelity. Her fears had only gotten more intense since starting therapy and as she continued to live with Ben over a longer period. Her accusations and questioning became more frequent, and Ben's patience waned. It seemed that Jennifer and Ben spent a disproportionate amount of time now arguing relative to time spent enjoying each other's company. Tension was mounting, and Jennifer continued to insist that this relationship was "her last chance."

In spite of this mounting tension, Jennifer's voice was steady in session. While she spoke about feeling anxious and constantly worried, I observed the inconsistency between her affect and the content of what she described. She could appear calm on the outside but on the inside she was a mess, spiraling out of control, and barely getting by. When I met Jennifer in the waiting room she appeared calm, collected, and almost jovial as we walked down the hallway. After she sat down in my office and we started talking, she quickly began to sob, fidgeting in her chair, with a lot of nervous gestures and movements. Jennifer was seemingly able to numb her emotions through substances and projective defenses. She denied her dependency needs until she became attached and dependent, at which point she felt out of control.

In our next session, I met the Jennifer she described internally. Perhaps I had given her permission by noticing the dissonance between what she said and what she revealed was truly happening. I went to greet her in the waiting room, and she sat, staring blankly ahead, her usual enthusiasm absent from her greeting. After a few minutes of silence in the consulting room, I asked Jennifer what she was thinking. She began to weep and said she had "f---ed everything up." She always "f---s everything up" and that she is "such a f---up" and "has been and always will be." I leaned in from my chair to let her know I was there with her and not afraid of her anger and distress. I calmly and gently nodded as she cried (more like wailing without tears) and expressed her self-hatred, all the while gesticulating as if pleading with someone.

When I asked what had happened she told me about a fight she had with Ben. He had been out, and Jennifer had become overwhelmed by her fears and mistrust while she was home alone. Upon his return, she demanded to know whom he had been with. I suggested that perhaps she wanted to escape the horrible emptiness and loneliness she was experiencing in the moment, and that while she was blaming herself for her actions, she was only trying to find a solution to her pain. I also suggested that she struggled with feeling alone and empty from an early age and she had been trying to find ways to escape that experience through substances and other methods but with limited success.

The idea that she was making great efforts at feeling better reassured Jennifer and quieted some of her self-loathing. She agreed that the need to escape these feelings of loneliness and self-loathing were familiar, but she seemed surprised that I linked these experiences to her early development. She said, "I didn't consider that before." She also had not connected her self-destructive efforts to avoidance before and this connection was an epiphany for her. "So my suicide attempt is similar to my accusations of Ben because I'm trying to cope with fears of abandonment? That's kinda crazy."

This reflection prompted Jennifer to wonder whether there was a better coping strategy for dealing with these downward ruminative spirals. I noticed her ego strength in those moments when I could interrupt her downward spirals by encouraging her to self-reflect with some compassion. I, too, experienced a sense of relief (in terms of my feeling of responsibility for her) as she met my efforts at promoting self-soothing with compassion toward herself. Jennifer was taking care of herself because I was modeling how to do this and giving her permission to practice. In this helpful caretaking, I could teach Jennifer to recognize why she was doing what she was doing and choose to act differently. I felt slightly less afraid of her projective efforts when I was able to identify things that were helpful and she responded to them. These moments of softening and improved self-regulation through reflection and perspective-taking were brief at first. They also were reminders to her of my presence. Sometimes, however, reminding her that I was there seemed to backfire, as she became afraid of losing me.

Jennifer left the climactic moment of her argument with Ben until the end of our session. If this relationship did not work out, she told me, she had vowed to kill herself. She stared at me when she said this, seemingly unaware of the gravity of what she was saying. This confession was during the 49th minute of the therapy hour, and she said she had also told this to Ben.

I asked her what it was like to say this to me. She reported that it was a relief that she had a plan if Ben broke up with her. She acknowledged that she felt less helpless with her feelings of abandonment and aloneness if she decided what she would do before they could overwhelm her. I suggested that her disclosing this to Ben (and later on to me) were efforts at keeping people close and trying to forestall abandonment. While she later admitted that she did not actually want to die, she reported she could not tolerate the experience of another failed romantic relationship or the prospect of even considering life with a new partner. She could not start over again.

Despite her efforts at reassuring me that she was not suicidal, I took Jennifer's comments seriously. She had a history of impulsivity, a previous suicide attempt, and was under a lot of distress. While I was careful not to react too strongly in the moment, I started our next meeting on this topic. We made a safety contract, discussed what she might do if she felt desperate again and tried to make concrete plans in terms of scheduling day-to-day activities. She had reportedly been isolating herself from her friends, and I encouraged her to reach out and spend time with them.

Over the course of the next 3 months Jennifer became more depressed and anxious and her relationship became more acrimonious. Our sessions felt like the movie *Groundhog Day*. Jennifer recounted episodes of her mistrust, a subsequent fight she had with Ben, and then her attempts at reconciling with him. The episodes of repair (after ruptures) seemed to be shorter in duration as treatment continued. Ben and Jennifer had more frequent fights and it seemed that Ben's frustration was amplifying as her fears were intensifying, and they were having difficulty returning to a state of equilibrium. As the relationship continued to deteriorate, Jennifer's episodes of paranoia became more frequent, and this manifested in the transference.

As in many training clinics, our sessions were audio taped, albeit de-identified. Jennifer had signed an informed consent at the start of treatment, but after a few months of therapy she became highly concerned about the taping. What happened to the recordings, who heard them, and did I listen to them and with whom? I was open and honest with these details and tried to explore Jennifer's fears. She denied being afraid and defensively justified her concerns as "normal" and challenged me by asking, "Would [you] want people listening to [your] deepest concerns?"

The nature of our relationship changed from collaborative and somewhat mature to more regressed and aggressive (seemingly paralleling her relationship with Ben) when Jennifer came to our next session telling me she was going to tape our meetings. She felt it was only "fair" for her to listen to me if I was listening to her. I was caught off guard and she was insistent about her efforts. She suggested that maybe she had been taping our meetings all along and maybe she would get more out of our therapy if she could "study" me and what had been said.

What if she had been taping me? In a flash moment, I imagined a posting on a social media site (YouTube or Facebook) with a career-ending critique of my abilities and competencies as a therapist, followed by a recording. This paranoid thought may have been a form of countertransference or projective identification. As these thoughts floated through my mind, I wondered if Jennifer could see the fear on my face. I reassured myself with some reality-testing and knew on some level that I needed to be present for this important moment and mindfully brought myself back in to the room.

I was resolute about her not taping and later understood these instincts as my concern about her becoming obsessional about our relationship, replaying the tape repeatedly, and dissecting what was said and what was not said, in a way that was not likely to be adaptive and would distract us from the intensity of our moment-to-moment relationship. I brought these ideas up to her at our next meeting, but she did not appear interested. "I was just curious," she said. It seemed the moment had passed or she had not really had the intention of taping in the first place.

I also started to wonder, at times, if twice weekly psychotherapy was too much or not enough for Jennifer. Was it possible that opening Jennifer up to her fears caused further destabilization? Perhaps she needed a slower pace and less intensity, and meeting with me twice weekly made her more exposed, similar to the way that she felt more vulnerable when she moved into the apartment with Ben. Conversely, I also wondered if Jennifer needed more therapy. While she did not voice this specifically, it might be possible that Jennifer felt unable to sustain the loss of only seeing me twice a week, and more frequent meetings would promote greater safety and stability for her. Or perhaps she needed a different approach—a more structured treatment focusing on affect regulation and other attempts at skill building. While I held these questions in mind, I used the process and content of our sessions to inform and continue the approach we were taking.

I felt she was using the therapy effectively to navigate the confusing, painful, and shameful experiences stirred up by her fragile attachments. Our alliance was strong and she was tolerating her pain in other areas of her life. She was maintaining both her jobs, had not relapsed on substances, and was consistently attending sessions and processing between meetings what we discussed, even though the pace had slowed down a bit. While the transference was becoming intense and would further intensify, she seemed to tolerate our work well enough to continue.

To augment the treatment, I recommended that Jennifer get a psychopharmacology consult as her mood and anxiety worsened. While she had initially been opposed to this idea, she was now more willing to consider a consult. As she felt with me when starting psychotherapy, Jennifer was initially ambivalent about describing her symptoms of distress to the psychiatrist, downplaying her anxiety and then feeling misunderstood. The psychiatrist and I stayed in close communication during the treatment to address these complexities.

The second phase of our work began several months into treatment when Jennifer's romantic relationship deteriorated further and she started to develop a more anxious attachment to me. Ben and Jennifer were talking about ending their relationship because of the problems they were having. They were still living together and trying to work things out, but their fights were more frequent and more vicious. I suggested to Jennifer during one of our sessions that she had been so afraid of being left that it appeared she had not considered how she felt about her relationship with Ben and how it was going. She did not elaborate on this idea during the session but in a subsequent meeting she said she had not considered how Ben was sometimes not the right partner for her. She could temporarily mobilize and consider whether she was not just afraid of Ben leaving, but afraid of her own desires to leave Ben. She could hold on to this dialectic for moments before coming back to her own fears of rejection.

Jennifer began to leave messages between sessions for me. She noted things she wanted to discuss on the voicemail. She said, for example, "I had been thinking about what you said about X, and that we should talk more about it next time." But, she said there was no need to call her back. I saw these messages as attempts at staying connected and attached to me between our meetings, and also noticed that I started to have to usher her out of sessions by standing up and reminding her that we were out of time. She often brought up topics at the end of sessions that seemed to invite more in-depth conversation.

Jennifer also revealed that she wondered about me. She wondered what I was like outside of sessions, what my friends were like, and what

I did for fun. She was curious if I was the "calm, loving, and under-standing" person I was in therapy with other people in my life. She won-dered if we had met under different circumstances whether we would be friends. I noticed comparisons between Ben and myself and Jennifer's wish that Ben would understand her better. She reported that in a recent argument she had told Ben she wished he was more like me and that he could "see the good in me like you." Her idealization of me seemed to be developing, and it was becoming clear that we would need plenty of time to process and plan for our ending. She was going to need to feel and express negative feelings toward me alongside these positive ones, and it would be important to help her integrate these opposing feelings.

The timing felt unfortunate because her romantic relationship was at a crisis point, and she and Ben were actively discussing breaking up. Remarkably, in the face of this emotional upheaval with Ben, her para-noia had lessened, and she was able to tolerate the anxiety that accompa-nied her fearful thoughts and even offer herself some perspective-taking ("Is there any evidence that this is true other than the intense feelings?"). Furthermore, she was engaged in treatment and we started actively dis-cussing our upcoming ending. I felt she was poised to do this critical work and we had laid an important foundation to do it together.

TERMINATION

In the third phase of the treatment, Jennifer's idealization of me deterio-rated as I reminded her about our impending termination. I described the termination process matter-of-factly at first, and we discussed her difficulties with endings and her fear of abandonment. I suggested that our ending was an opportunity, as painful as it might be, for us to work with these anxieties more closely and for her to have control in how we said good-bye even if it was not entirely on her own terms. We predicted her ambivalence at wanting to come to future sessions, her likely feelings of desperation, and her fears of planning for a future without me.

Although Jennifer received the reminder of our termination calmly, I feared that she would descend into rageful threats of suicide. In the next session, Jennifer was more irritable than I had ever experienced her, coming in to the session late (e.g., "Oh, I hardly noticed the time—guess it was later than I thought.") cutting me off frequently and deriding my attempts at interpretation. Most disconcertingly, she seemed to enjoy my growing sense of confusion and frustration as I struggled to find ways to communicate and connect to her without constantly being rejected and rebuked myself. At one point, I confessed to her that it seemed nothing I said was quite right and I had the impression that no matter what I said, she might be upset with it. She smiled at this, told me I just "wasn't getting it," and acted unfazed by my observation or by any of her behaviors and their affect on the therapy. I understood Jennifer's anger as an attempt to get me to reject her but also as an effort at punishing me for leaving. She could not make use of these ideas when I brought them up, and either minimized their significance or rejected them altogether. I felt it was important to continue bringing to her awareness fears of my leaving and her rage at my abandonment. I was pleased that she felt safe and trusting enough to be willing to share this anger with me, even if it was via passive–aggressive and not fully conscious expressions. She was experiencing and communicating about her loss differently and I was proud of her efforts.

I encouraged Jennifer to talk about her anger at termination and tried to gently prompt her by commenting, "I could imagine you'd be mad at me for leaving our therapy before we are finished" and "I imagine you may want to miss our sessions and punish me for leaving you by leaving me first." Much to her credit, Jennifer only missed one session during this difficult termination process. She cried for the first time in therapy about her many "lost" relationships and the lonely feelings she carried around with her. She came late to several sessions but she showed up.

I was also experiencing Jennifer differently and did not feel as frustrated or angry. I could empathize with her conflict and fears of abandonment more vividly as she openly discussed it and we lived through it together. There was more directness and less projective identification. I was deeply moved by her courage and resilience during this stage of treatment and related this to her. She nodded in acknowledgment, and we both knew she was experiencing this loss differently by being able to tolerate my leaving and not leaving before me or feeling flooded with anxiety. While I told her I wished I could continue this work with her, I was also confident she would be able to translate our experience into other interpersonal relationships with confidence about her own abilities.

During the termination period, she and Ben made the decision to end their relationship. Jennifer did not make any efforts or threats of suicide. She did not relapse into substance use. She maintained employment and found a room she could rent at a friend's apartment. She did not pursue efforts, however, at finding a new therapy relationship despite my encouragement and referrals. Jennifer continued to wonder about me during the termination—where did I shop for my clothes, what drink did I order at Starbucks, and did I have a boyfriend? The questions felt less like idealization or attempts at merger (i.e., she did not seem to be requesting answers, just wondered aloud with me to witness them) and more like overtures and attempts at trying to know who I was as a separate person.

She came to our last session directly from work, perspiring and out of breath from riding her skateboard. I could not help but recall her early memory of saving up to buy her skateboard and wanting her parents to delight in her efforts. As I came to know Jennifer, I saw more of this young girl who was quieted, rejected, and shamed. When we shook hands at our last session, she was willing to tolerate the grief and pain she witnessed and experienced throughout her life, represented by her ability to tolerate her loss of our relationship.

Through the therapy, we started to weave an internal net of self-regulation, affect tolerance, compassion, and forgiveness, which meant that she would not inevitably fall into despair and feel overwhelmed when faced with loss. Jennifer was no longer a victim to her own impulses and intense affective states. She could still experience her feelings but with the security of knowing that she could get through them. I hoped and believed that with continued treatment and her own efforts Jennifer would continue to engage in relationships and her life more maturely as an independent adult.

ASSESSMENT OF PROGRESS

Organizing Jennifer's complex clinical presentation around the core dynamic theme of fear of abandonment was challenging yet useful in many ways. In the recitation of her anxieties, Jennifer announced her fear of abandonment at the outset of treatment. It was therefore critical to maintain a view of the treatment's end in order to predict and intervene with her possible fragmentation in the face of losing her relationship with me. The clearest instance of Jennifer's treatment gains was her ability to survive the end of her relationship with Ben as well as the end of our treatment relationship. Rather than falling apart as these relationships ended, Jennifer maintained a frame for herself—a home and a job—which was no small feat for this self-described wanderer. Overall, Jennifer exceeded my expectations in terms of enduring the losses of two intense relationships without severe regression or internal disintegration. I could have easily been mistaken by Jennifer's initial presentation, in terms of understanding her level of functioning. Similarly, I could have underestimated the amount of work it would require to help her with the emotions associated with this termination. I have wondered how Jennifer has internalized our relationship and her experiences in treatment. What happened the days and weeks after our final session? I sometimes found myself looking at skateboarders in the neighborhood wondering if one could be Jennifer, or smiling at the sight of these riders with memories of her development and efforts in treatment.

When I began treating Jennifer I was fearful of my ability to provide psychodynamic therapy with someone who had difficulties with reality testing. At times, I felt pulled to do more behavioral interventions (especially with the threat of suicidal thinking and degree of affective flooding) and "rescue" Jennifer from her own pain. I frequently brought these conflicts to supervision and tried to understand my motivation to be more prescriptive in treatment, and worked on understanding the transferential experiences and enactments that may have contributed to these impulses. In moments of being more prescriptive I may have been motivated by my own fears of the intensity of Jennifer's emotions instead of trying to help her tolerate these feelings, which ultimately was extremely important for her own growth and internal stability. In using my ability to tolerate and withstand Jennifer's disavowed anxieties, overwhelming feelings and rage, I modeled a capacity for emotion regulation. In doing so, I was able to counter Jennifer's efforts at confirming her feelings of badness and unworthiness. I allowed her to work through the range of her feelings from rage to grief, without reenacting the rejections she had so frequently experienced.

My growth paralleled Jennifer's: as she learned to tolerate the range of her affects, I learned (and am learning) to tolerate and make productive use of my countertransference. At times, I wondered how I could have made greater use of my countertransference in trying to help Jennifer—for example, to help her understand Ben's reactions to her, or to help her understand her reactions to herself. I hesitated in these moments because I thought it was better for her to experience her own affects, and also because I feared she might disintegrate into paranoia. I am aware, however, I may have made different choices in such moments with Jennifer had I known then what I know now.

Jennifer's future work is in developing the ability to trust within active, intimate relationships—to survive her fears of abandonment, and to accept, own, and reduce her tendency to enact the fears that have fueled her patterns that undermined previous relationships. At the end of our work together, she was attempting to obtain private medical insurance and was compliant with the psychiatric medications she had been prescribed. I hope she continued to pursue both therapy and psychopharmacology. I often wonder how Jennifer is doing, especially because we had to end early, and also because I was impressed with the amount of internal change that happened during a relatively brief but intense psychotherapy. I believe she will be able to use her positive experiences from our relationship to risk being in therapy again.

CHAPTER 9

"I CAN'T LEAVE HIM, I THINK HE LOVES ME"

A Case of Fear of Abandonment

ROBERT SCHWEITZER
ALIX VANN

Kate is a chaotic, abandonment-sensitive young woman who entered treatment to get help with her relationship problems, emotional lability, and feelings of emptiness. The therapist provided a safe container for Kate's complex and conflicted feelings while at the same time allowing for a discussion of those emotions. She maintained a balance between open-ended exploration, support, and clear boundaries for the patient.

Through the case history, and in the personal reflections at the end, the therapist is articulate about her observations about herself, the patient, and the treatment. These observations become important data for her in conceptualizing the treatment and making decisions about which techniques to implement. The associated observations by the therapist's supervisor are particularly meaningful and enrich the case, as it is rare to have access to the supervisor's perspective in a case history.

There are several interesting issues brought up by this case history. First, helping patients who are involved in pathologic relationships requires helping them see what is really going on and supporting their healthy choices, but maintaining reasonable expectations—people cannot change too much or too fast. The therapist had to work hard to keep her expectations appropriately in check. Second, recreational drug use and addiction clearly interfered with the impact of therapy, and it is a challenge to decide how and when to address this to allow for meaningful work to continue. Third, objective assessment provides an important counterbalance to the therapist's perception of progress and is especially important for patients with multiple problems any one of which could be the entire focus of a treatment. Finally, outside consultation for patients who stir up particularly intense countertransference experiences is invaluable for regaining an overall sense of perspective.

We were walking back from the tram after celebrating our ninth month together. The weather was overcast with that Melbourne grey. Kate was attired in her usual black top, black jeans, black Doc Martens, with jet black hair worn over her face. I asked her about her day. "The bastard always makes me do the dirty work. I was cleaning tables till after 4:00. My shift finishes at 3:00. Why does he always do this to me?" Everyone was unfair to Kate. She asked me about my day. "Good enough!" I was not sure her mind was on me. We got into our apartment, and she started up with it again. "I'm feeling bad again. Things are getting bad." She always tells me how bad she feels. She predicts that I will leave her and that our relationship is doomed, yet she wants me to make things better, like a little girl wanting to be cared for. I told her that I was sick of trying to reason with her, when she again started throwing her phone against the wall. "You are always thinking about yourself. You never think about me. Why won't you just listen to me? Yet another phone smashed! I have heard it so many times: I need you; I need you to fix it!" Her voice got louder and I felt increasingly impotent. She came at me, and I feared the worst. I lifted my arm, grabbed her and bundled her up. This seems to be the only way I can control her. Holding her, and drugging her. I did not know which she preferred! It can't go on. I resolved to seek professional help for Kate.

—KEN, NOTE FROM A JOURNAL

CHIEF COMPLAINT AND PRESENTATION

Ken is a guitarist with a small-time urban band. "I need you to see Kate." With these words, Ken referred his partner, Kate, to our clinic. As part of the referral, he provided the excerpt from his journal we reprinted above.

Kate entered the first session with some trepidation. She presented as a petite young woman with fine features and dyed black hair, which she wore in dreadlocks. She was neatly groomed, and wore a black dress, black cardigan, and black eye makeup, which contributed to an intense, gothic-like appearance, significantly younger than her stated age of 21. She was of small stature, often sitting forward and responsive to questions. She appeared familiar with the process of therapy, as she spoke softly and thoughtfully about her history and the reasons for her coming to therapy. Her very first words were, "Ken wants me to come here."

Kate described chronic feelings of emptiness, a "gaping hole inside" her, guilt, and a sense that she was a bad person. She spoke of oscillating between thinking these feelings were legitimate and feeling unjustified in feeling anything. She described a constant sense of angst and panic. As we discussed her feelings in more specific detail, she said she felt "radioactive" and unable to "let people be really close." She described being presently "the most sober" she had been in the last 2 years, which was "not nice," but that she was still smoking marijuana daily as well as taking a variety of prescription drugs, procured for her by Ken. Kate was working full-time at an inner city cafe and dreaded going to work every day, saying it felt like she was a "little girl" and people would always "pick on" her. Kate felt increasingly isolated in her relationship with Ken, but said she knew he was "jealous and controlling" out of love for her—whatever he did was "for her own good."

HISTORY

Kate is the older of two daughters. Until she was 12 years old, when her parents separated, Kate said she had had a "great" upbringing. During the first session, she described her mother as being the "perfect Mum" who was involved in playgroups and often had other children over to play. She described Mum as engaging and wanting the best for her, with an underlying competitiveness. Over time, she described feeling quite overwhelmed by her mother and also fearful in relation to her inability to always make Mum happy. Her father was easygoing and passive—the opposite of her mother. She recalled her Dad supporting her academically within the school environment and valuing more intellectual pursuits, but felt he abandoned her to fend for herself when it came to her mother. Kate revealed a sense of being "different" from the time she was young. While her sister was "normal," Kate was "morose" and sad.

Kate remembered biting a girl on the face on her first day of playgroup so that the girl's face bled. By the age of 5, once she had started school, Kate felt lonely, isolated, and "yucky," walking around the playground alone. As she moved into grades three and four, Kate became more popular and confident. She dominated the other children and was the "bossy leader" of her peer group. Toward the end of grade four and into grade five, Kate described intense feelings of isolation and "nothingness." Things "fell apart" in grade five. Kate had no friends, she ate lunch with the teachers, and she engaged in self-destructive behavior. As she described it, she would get into the bathtub and "cut [my]self up." Kate sensed that there must be something about her that made her worthy of the hate she felt from the other children in her school, and yet she was never able to understand why she felt so rejected. She thought she must have been "really annoying."

Kate's 12th year was tumultuous. That year, her father was diagnosed with a brain tumor and given 1 month to live. Kate remembers feeling guilty for not feeling sad enough for her father. However, after an operation he "miraculously survived" and is still alive today. Kate's parents separated soon after her father was discharged from the hospital and Kate recalled wondering whether her mother may have been having an affair at this time. Kate and her sister both lived with their mother following the separation.

Kate found herself in relationships, often with young males, in which she felt used, put down, and felt fortunate to be noticed. When she was just 15 years old she met a boy who appeared to have everything going for him within his own family of origin. At the same time, she experienced her mother as being inaccessible and unavailable. Kate recalled significant conflict with her mother around the same age, often revolving around her mother's wish to set limits and Kate experiencing her mother as overly controlling and distrustful. These conflicts resulted in her being kicked out of home. Kate stated with some disdain that her mother's version of the story was that Kate ran away.

She left home to live with her new boyfriend and his family. As the story unfolded, Kate revealed the degree to which she became a "servant" in his home. She was given house duties, and ended up being a surrogate nanny for a younger daughter within the family, leading to further experiences of feeling used. It appeared that there was so much that was expected of her and never discussed, that she simply fell into the role of doing what was required. Kate's boyfriend and his mother were regular drug users, and they were happy to share their supplies with Kate. She started smoking marijuana, and this soon escalated into other drugs including cocaine and Ecstasy.

Kate experimented with both sex and drugs on an almost daily basis. Just as her drug experiences provided her with relief from her sense of self, her sexual experiences were literally at the hands of her partner, who made all kinds of demands to which she succumbed. Some of these involved engaging with him sexually in public arenas, during which she may or may not have been observed. However, the common theme was that all of these encounters were about the needs of her partner, with little consideration of her own feelings. Nevertheless, these experiences stood out as being positive for Kate, as she stated she liked sex and felt comforted by it. She recalled being initially frightened, but this soon gave way to a sense of relief from her own tortured sense of self.

After 2 years, the level of abuse within her boyfriend's home became intolerable. Furthermore, Kate reported a member of the family for child neglect, which made it impossible for her to continue living with the family. She packed her bags and moved in with another young man who had shown an interest in her, "Mr. Über Cool." He was thoughtful, showed some sensitivity, and was in love with her. He was also tolerant of her drug habits and happy to facilitate whatever she wanted. The more she got to know him, the more thoughtful and sensitive he appeared to be. She described a recurring pattern. The more Mr. Über Cool provided her with opportunities to express herself, the more anxious Kate became that she "did not belong to him" and thus questioned their relationship. She recalls experiencing him as a "wimp." For some reason, the ideas of love, possession, power, and ownership seemed to be juxtaposed in Kate's mind. Kate experienced his not trying to control her as a reflection of her not being "special" enough. How could this man be good for her if he let her "get away with anything"?

Over time, Kate described spending more time with another man, Ken, who procured drugs on demand. Her relationship with Ken became more intense. At the time she wondered how Mr. Über Cool could tolerate her spending time with Ken. She concluded that he could not love her sufficiently to allow her this freedom. When Kate finally decided that she had no choice but to leave Mr. Über Cool, Ken was happy to take her in. Within a week, Ken had confessed his love for Kate and promised that if she stayed with him, he would take care of her better than anyone else ever had. Kate and Ken have been living together in an intimate relationship since this time, and this relationship has also been turbulent.

CORE PSYCHODYNAMIC PROBLEM AND FORMULATION
Part I: Summarizing Statement

Kate is a 21-year-old woman currently working full-time as a waitress at an inner-city cafe. She was referred by her live-in boyfriend who had previously been her drug dealer. She described constantly feeling bad and guilty, a sense of emptiness and loneliness, a history of self-destructive behavior with suicide ideation, and reported a history of tumultuous relationships. She presents as a fragile young woman with significant self-destructive patterns, including drug and alcohol use, and is motivated to gain some understanding of both herself and others. She describes a feeling of "stuckness" in her current life pattern with little ability to trust her own experiences and feelings.

Part II: Description of Nondynamic Factors

Kate described herself as a shy and difficult child. Her temperament was brittle as she struggled with interpersonal relationships with both her mother and peers. Kate has had contact with psychiatrists from the age of 12, seemingly as a result of difficulties within her home and because of her mother's anxiety in responding to Kate's outbursts. She described her previous therapy as comprising learning anxiety management techniques and medication in the form of venlafaxine (Effexor), which she did not find useful. Kate had never attended therapy for more than twelve sessions, and her mother reportedly sabotaged therapy when it was implied that she might have played a role in Kate's experiences.

From the age of 15, she has taken illicit substances such as Ecstasy, cocaine, marijuana, and combinations of these. Kate had a period of alcohol abuse at age 20, drinking up to three bottles of wine a day. She uses a variety of prescription drugs, mainly oxycontin, Xanax, and codeine, with marijuana daily. She reported her intake of these is increasing as she develops tolerance.

Currently, Kate resides with her partner, who provides her with prescription drugs. She describes having little autonomy within her relationship with him.

Part III: Psychodynamic Explanation of Central Conflicts

Kate's core psychodynamic problem is fear of abandonment with an associated fragmented sense of self and unstable object relations. Her main conflicts involve her fragile sense of self, feelings of badness and guilt, and issues around dependency and attachment. My hypothesis is that Kate experienced limited emotional containment from a young age due to the lack of a relationship with her primary attachment figure, her mother, and this made it difficult for her to integrate the different aspects of herself and develop her own mentalizing abilities [that is, the ability to understand oneself as a coherent whole person with mixed thoughts and feelings, relating to others who have a similar subjective experience and emotional makeup (Bateman & Fonagy, 2006)].

There appears to have been an early rupture in the relationship between Kate and her mother, as Kate's mother may have had a similarly limited ability to self-regulate and mentalize, which may have resulted in Kate internalizing her mother as a bad, damaging object. Kate's conflictual and emotionally tumultuous relationship with her mother may have affected her ability to develop a stable sense of self. The lack of an unconditional loving, soothing, and mirroring experience with her mother probably made it difficult for Kate to develop sufficient self-soothing capacities and thus the ability to internalize and contain the more aggressive, destructive aspects of her self.

Similarly, Kate may have had difficulty in experiencing validation, recognition, and a sense of mutuality in the eyes of her father, whom she described as "passive" and "emotionally unavailable." The lack of early attunement resulting from attachment problems with both parents resulted in Kate feeling lonely and abandoned. This may also have left Kate feeling anger toward her parents, particularly her mother, along with intense guilt and badness about such feelings.

Two vignettes illustrate this psychodynamic conceptualization. First, Kate recalled vivid memories of the ongoing conflict between her parents, their lack of awareness of her needs and how this made it hard for her to understand her own needs and develop a mind of her own. Kate recalled feeling anxious about an upcoming second-grade math test and being unable to sleep. Crying and shaking, she recalls trying to approach each of her parents for help. They were overly concerned with their own issues and paid little attention to Kate's needs at that time. Her mother dismissed her, telling her she was just being silly, and her father passively went along with this. Despite his passivity, Kate felt that her father was the only figure who provided her with any support at this time, as opposed to her mother whom she perceived as competitive and critical. Consequently, when her parents separated and her father left, Kate experienced a deep sense of loss accompanied by some empathy for her mother's distress.

On some level, Kate also felt blamed for her father leaving the family home, and for the dissolution of at least one of her mother's subsequent romantic relationships. Following this, her mother had relationships with men which were at times tumultuous and, in at least one case, Kate felt blamed for the dissolution of a relationship which her mother had valued. However, Kate's lack of memory for any incidents during her early childhood is a striking feature of her presentation. My hypothesis is that her intense feelings of abandonment led her to repress these painful experiences.

In a second vignette, Kate left home when she was just 15 to live with her boyfriend with whom she was madly in love. As previously mentioned, the relationship was highly destructive, as the boyfriend was sexually abusive and his parents were emotionally abusive. She described a passive acceptance of her role within the adopted family and engagement in increasingly self-destructive behaviors, including significant drug use.

The Core Conflictual Relationship Theme (CCRT) for Kate is that she wishes to be acknowledged, understood, and taken care of, but feels that others abandon her or try to control her. Kate responds to others by feeling bad and guilty, and reacts by becoming dependent and passive, or acting out through verbal outbursts and self-harming behavior. These issues are reflected in Kate's ongoing drug use and her continued engagement in a relationship that is potentially destructive. These two vignettes and their reflection in the CCRT illustrate Kate's early dysfunctional relational experiences. Such experiences, combined with her continued experience of tumultuous relationships, may well have contributed to her fragmented and fragile sense of self. As a result, she experiences chronic anxiety, which she describes as a "panicky feeling," in the context of her relationships. She defends against anxiety and feelings of powerlessness and vulnerability through primitive mechanisms such as regression, splitting, and projection, and is functioning at a borderline level.

Kate continues to use drugs and act out self-destructively toward herself and others. For example, during the therapy there have been several violent arguments with Ken which resulted in Kate grabbing Ken, and one in which she also smashed her mobile phone in the process. This behavior is consistent with her fear of developing an attachment with another for fear of abandonment, and the maladaptive ways in which she attempts to control her aggressive impulses. She acts out to deal with her conflicted feelings, and this dysfunctional behavior, in turn, creates more stress and anxiety. The absence of positive relationships diminishes her opportunity to gain a different experience of herself. Her poor attachment experiences may intensify her already vulnerable attachment system, resulting in acute distress.

Kate's sense that there is a different way to experience relationships, her ability to know her limits in some settings, and her hope for the future have helped her cope so far. Kate has shown a certain amount of resilience, particularly when she presented for her regular session several days after a self-admission to a hospital emergency department.

Kate's difficulties occur against a family history that includes her mother with impulse control problems and her father's passivity. There was also family conflict leading to the early separation of her parents. The parental impulsivity suggests the possibility that Kate has a biological vulnerability to borderline functioning. It is likely that her consistent use of drugs to manage these difficult experiences may also be reinforcing her sense of isolation within relationships.

Part IV: Predicting Responses to the Therapeutic Situation

The therapy will aim at serving a containing function for Kate's high levels of distress. This in itself may provide a corrective experience for Kate as she may not have experienced containment in previous significant relationships. Part of the therapeutic process will also involve a focus on supporting Kate's strengths, without fostering a regressive dependent relationship. Kate may attempt to push the limits of the therapeutic relationship due to her fear of abandonment, so it will be important to work within a stable frame while being responsive to Kate's needs.

Following the development of an initial positive therapeutic relationship, Kate's internal splitting may become reflected in the transference, such that she alternately idealizes and devalues me. This fluctuation will reflect Kate's internal struggle between dependency and abandonment, and awareness of countertransference will be important to avoid enactments.

Though Kate appears to have significant ego weakness, as evidenced by her impaired judgment and apparent difficulty persisting with relationships, she also appears to be motivated to understand how her past has affected her present and to achieve some sense of autonomy. It is likely that the process of therapy may initially be difficult for Kate, as she is used to feeling misunderstood. She may act out in therapy in an attempt to recreate the relational pattern with which she is familiar. A therapeutic stance of neutrality and supportiveness will therefore be important, and potential enactments may be used to interpret transference, repair the rupture, and provide a consistent and continuous other who can be trusted. In this way, Kate may have the opportunity to internalize a healthier relational pattern that may allow her to develop a more stable sense of self.

COURSE OF TREATMENT

In describing the treatment, I will refer to four phases: the initial phase where I focused on gaining a better understanding of Kate, developing a working bond and providing containment in response to Kate's significant level of distress; an intensification of the transferential relationship; a crisis which contributed to Kate's and my reflecting more deeply on our relationship; and finally, an "awareness" phase during which Kate began to gain a greater understanding of herself in relation to both me and her partner. This phase was also associated with greater uncertainties which were not resolved.

During the early phase of therapy, Kate talked in a somewhat detached manner as she described her relationship with her partner and her family of origin. She often described events in her life, the mundane nature of her job, and her dependence upon her partner. She made occasional reference to her use of drugs. During those weeks she often spoke about conflict with Ken. She showed limited interest in focusing on her inner life, but instead gave the impression of being dependent and "help-seeking."

Kate described a high degree of psychic pain, as evidenced in the ongoing assessment of her functioning (see her Outcome Questionnaire 45 [OQ-45] scores in the "Assessment of Progress" section). An early therapeutic goal was to provide Kate with a sense of comfort in being with herself and a greater understanding of the subtle and complex shifts in her mood, within a safe environment. This process involved a range of techniques, such as exploration of past experiences, memories, thoughts, and fantasies. Often I helped her to get in touch with previously unexpressed affects, particularly as they related to early relationships. She was resistant to exploring early parental experiences during this phase.

The intensity of Kate's painful feelings was often overwhelming for her. A core early process in therapy related to helping her to contain her feelings. Her distress was based both within a historical context and in her current living arrangement. Recalling early adolescent experiences allowed previously warded off emotions to emerge. However, the emergence of such emotions also escalated her difficulties rather than provided her with healing. The only way I could help Kate contain these experiences was to guide her to explore such feelings within the context of a positive working alliance and to support her capacity for soothing and self-awareness (Summers & Barber, 2010).

The development and maintenance of the therapeutic alliance was important and complex from the beginning of therapy. In the first session, Kate mentioned that she had tried therapy several times before but had never found it very successful. In reflecting on the first six sessions of therapy, Kate said she felt that things had been getting worse in general, but that she was finding coming to therapy and "talking things through" to be useful and "cathartic." Kate was also quick to say this attempt at therapy was "working better than anything else ever had." It seemed Kate was able to experience a connection with me during the early phase, and despite her sense that other aspects of her internal and external life were worsening, she now had someone in her corner.

Just as Kate appeared to develop a bond with me early on, I too found myself powerfully aligned with Kate. Her palpable vulnerability evoked a therapeutic response in me that made me want to address her immediate needs. At the same time, I knew I needed to appropriately monitor the issues being presented and maintain an analytic stance, which balanced Kate's need for structure and responsiveness. I saw my task as facilitating her sense of curiosity. I also was aware I was pressuring myself to be a good enough therapist to a patient my own age. I experienced her level of self-destructiveness as difficult to contain and deal with therapeutically. There was always the temptation to go into a "problem-solving" mode which would have been motivated by my own anxiety and a feeling that the therapy was not going anywhere. Supervision became increasingly important in assisting me to tolerate the painful affect which I experienced during my work with Kate.

In the next phase of treatment, the emotional intensity of the therapeutic relationship greatly increased. During the latter part of the second month of therapy, I sensed a more intense transference reaction and similarly a significant degree of countertransference. Kate sat down and shared the degree to which she felt out of control. Kate increasingly spoke to me as if I were her confidant, sharing things she could not say to anyone else, and telling me her deepest fears about her relationship with Ken. Perhaps I was becoming an idealized mother. In turn, I felt increasingly hostile to her partner which, I was aware, would not be helpful to Kate. At the same time I felt increasingly protective of Kate.

She seemed so vulnerable and isolated, a theme that would emerge in many of her relational episodes, and I wondered whether this sense of vulnerability would come to characterize our relationship too—something that, as a newer therapist, made me feel timid to use exploratory techniques such as interpretation. I was concerned that Kate was becoming more vulnerable as she sensed my availability and desire to help.

Kate recalled a recurring dream during this phase of the therapy. When she was just 6 or 7 years old, she dreamt she was in her original house and her parents left to go out. She was left with a woman who is a friend of her parents, but who is actually her Mum. She and this "Mum" were in the toy room, and Kate noticed that "Mum" was quite deformed, almost as if something was "mentally wrong" with her. "Mum" was unable to speak properly, had a shaved head with spiky bits of hair regrowing, was bloated and bigger than in real life, hunched over, and naked. Kate felt scared and repulsed by this woman. "Mum" pulled the skin off one side of her face. Kate knew that this woman was capable of doing this, so she was not surprised. "Mum" chased her around the toy room in circles, trying to bite Kate, biting her in the flesh of her back and shoulders, and holding the half of her face she had peeled off in one hand.

When exploring the meaning of the dream, Kate said, "I guess she killed me," though the dream always ended when Kate was being bitten and chased around the room. Kate's association and expansion of the dream images suggested that she thought the dream was about Mum being "a scary thing" whom Kate was being "left alone with." As Kate identified with the dream images, she described feeling separate when her Mum and Dad left her in the dream, and a palpable fear in being left alone with her Mum. She felt like she "didn't want it [Mum] to touch me because it was like she was diseased." Similarly, she recalled the toy room as big, cold, hard, and dark.

In working with Kate to make sense of the recurring themes in her dream, I noted the ambiguity of the images. The images seemed to fuse both good and bad aspects, which on one level, seemed related to her mother. But, I also thought that on an intrapsychic level, these images reflected her own psychic processes. That is, although her parents could be capable of being supportive they were also destructive, to the point where she experienced her mother as scary and monstrous.

If one takes the view that dream images often reflect one's own sense of self or split off aspects of herself, the dream raised questions about the degree to which Kate needed to deal with aspects of her self which she experienced as abhorrent and untouchable. The primitive images in the dream material suggested that therapy had a long way to go before Kate would be able to feel comfortable with and integrate these aspects of self.

I found myself appreciating her level of desperation and sadness, and her labile emotion filled all the space in the room as she covered these difficult issues. I felt a strong desire to be the one to save Kate from these experiences, to make a difference when no one before had been able to. However, I also had a sense for the first time that my relationship with Kate left me feeling empty, as if everything was being taken out of me and I was getting nothing back. I struggled with this feeling and also wondered whether Kate had any appreciation of what she was putting me through. There was so much emptiness and desolation present that it made me wonder whether there was even more early trauma or severe attachment difficulty with her mother than Kate was able to remember.

Reflecting upon my own countertransference feelings of both emptiness and the urge to rescue, it was almost like helping a bird with a broken wing that was utterly and desperately dependent upon me, and yet does not want to be touched by me. There were times where I felt intimately connected with Kate and at the same time I felt that any approach would be countenanced by immediate rejection. When I raised the issue of the clinic closing over the end-of-year break, her response was: "Oh, that's OK, I haven't really thought about it. I try not to think about it. And anyway, soon you will leave and be off doing this for real." I recognized the degree to which she felt both dependent and potentially abandoned.

In the next phase of therapy, a few months into the treatment, Kate regressed and there was a behavioral crisis that led me to reflect upon our relationship. The crisis was ostensibly associated with her sister being diagnosed with a significant illness. However, the timing of this crisis, at a time when the alliance was palpably deepening, made me wonder whether the crisis was also in part a response to her increased awareness of her use of drugs to mask her difficulties and her sense of isolation. Kate engaged in some acute self-harming behavior, including a drug overdose. This behavior was accompanied by suicidal ideation and an explosive argument with her partner, and she was briefly hospital-ized.

During this period, however, Kate did not miss a session. She was extremely distressed and commenced antidepressant medication. It seemed she had been overwhelmed by her own capacity and potential for disintegration. The same week that she admitted herself to the hos-pital, Kate attended her session with me and said, "You're the closest thing I have to a friend." This reinforced my appreciation of the signifi-cance of our relationship for Kate, as well as her sense of isolation. I also pondered my capacity to live up to Kate's expectations. This was not a comfortable experience.

I became aware of the degree to which Kate was continuing to struggle. Her ongoing drug use and passivity contributed to her regres-sion and she seemed to struggle to have a separate sense of identity and volition. She wanted to be close but this felt like enmeshment to her, and she was scared about feeling independent because this made her feel lonely and scared. In reflecting on the therapy with my supervisor at this point, I began to recognize the degree to which I had identified with Kate and this made it challenging to be objective and separate enough to maintain my role as her therapist.

In the fourth and most recent phase of treatment, in the 3 months after the hospitalization, Kate seemed to be more open and trusting and she appeared to feel a little more secure herself. Two particular themes emerged. Kate became increasingly aware of me. She made such com-ments as, "I see that you have dyed your hair." It seemed that the crisis had somehow caused Kate to be more fully engaged in the therapy. Sig-nificantly, though, she began to express dissatisfaction with her partner, and for the first time she described him as controlling and wondered whether they could continue their relationship.

Kate appeared tentative as she expressed her doubts about the via-bility of her relationship. At the same time, she appeared to be engaging in a process of separation and individuation, both in relation to myself as her therapist, and also in her relationship with her partner. She was able to express negative feelings and attitudes about Ken and the dynamic of their relationship, and she was beginning to explore new friendships. She had been offered a new job, having successfully held her previous position for over a year, one of her longest employments to date. She was also tentatively forging connections with her new, female coworkers. All of these changes were significant given her history.

There was a part of me that wanted to express my delight with these changes, but I was cautious not to appear overly enthusiastic. I sensed that enthusiasm on my part could contribute to Kate retreating and potentially regressing as she sought to contain her anxieties. Many supervision sessions centered on the degree to which therapy should emphasize reassurance as opposed to being more challenging. However, gradually Kate and I were able to explore more adult and realistic perceptions of her current relationships, to understand these relationships in terms of past relationships, and to discover the necessity of new ways of relating based on a sense of autonomy and strength.

Despite having made gains in her awareness of her relationships with significant others, and of past relationships, Kate continued to feel quite lonely and isolated. Her use of drugs continued to some extent, and she was finding it difficult to translate insights she gained from the therapy into behavioral responses and making lasting changes in her life. Within the sessions she also struggled to access her emotional life, often looking to me for guidance on what she should talk about. She preferred to provide me with a chronicle of the week's events as opposed to sharing feelings. I sensed that she was afraid of exploring experiences too deeply.

Kate's previous and current use of drugs was perhaps a resistance, with Kate using these substances as a way to avoid that which was most painful to her. She had also commented on her previous use of sex as a way of avoiding facing up to her situation. It is noteworthy that one of her drugs of choice was oxycontin, a powerful opiate analgesic. Although I was always aware of Kate's drug use, it was perhaps an oversight on my part not to address her drug use more actively, and consider the potential impact her use was having on the therapy. Furthermore, I started to see Kate as using both intellectualization and rationalization as she sought to distance herself from her experiences and justify remaining in a relationship with me.

My feelings about Kate were complex. As she revealed her consistent level of distress, I continued feeling that I was giving a lot and yet she was not as responsive as I might have expected. I was aware that Kate had a fragile sense of self and wondered about my own capacities to continue to tolerate the stress that emerged during the sessions. Her sense of craziness was potentially infectious. I recall the importance of supervision and my own therapy, providing me with the resources to continue to work with Kate during this difficult time.

Psychotherapy has been described as "a series of moments of attachment and engagement" (Summers & Barber, 2010, p. 236). The therapy with Kate comprised such a series of moments. Our early work was characterized by both distance and commitment, and over time there were moments of intense closeness that were potentially anxiety-provoking

for both Kate and me. Kate did not take kindly to outwardly affirming statements and yet there were also moments of closeness in which
she and I appeared to share the experience of being two young women,
struggling with our identities and ourselves.

One's identity as a newer therapist is fragile, with its own ups and
downs. However, for Kate, identity issues appeared to be at the core
of her difficulties. Her fear of abandonment, together with the wish to
merge with me, were pivotal in understanding the significant moments
in Kate's therapy, as well as in the progress of the therapy to date.

ASSESSMENT OF PROGRESS

When Kate commenced therapy, her main concerns were her affective
lability and her current relationship with Ken. I used the OQ-45 assessment instrument to assess her week-by-week response to the treatment.
The OQ-45 is one of several newly developed measures that aim to
assess therapeutic response (Lambert, Lunnen, Umphress, Hansen, &
Burlingame, 1994). Kate's levels of distress on this measure were within
the extreme range and were comparable to those of an inpatient psychiatric population.

Over the first eight sessions her anxiety increased, reflected in
an increase in her scores on the OQ-45 instrument. It was not until
4 months into the therapy that she gradually began to evidence some
improvement in her OQ-45 scores (see Figure 9.1); however, they have
remained within an elevated range.

Over the past 9 months, Kate has had some significant improvement. She has maintained her job and she has been able to use the opportunity to get to know herself better and tolerate her feelings using the
therapeutic relationship more effectively. She has begun to question her
role in relationships. She has shown initiative in reaching out to others, and most recently has talked about engaging in further study and
pursuing an independent career. She continues to be highly distressed,
experiencing conflict in her relationship with her partner, but is also able
to reflect upon these experiences and her own role in the genesis of such
conflict. She appears to have a better sense of the future, which may
involve some degree of independence as well as interdependence with
members of her family. While she would not be regarded as recovered
using traditional criteria, her current functioning suggests that she will
continue to be able to utilize the resources provided through the therapy,
and gain a greater sense of wholeness and personal integrity.

The continuing goals for therapy include working collaboratively
to gain further resolution of some of her family of origin-related issues

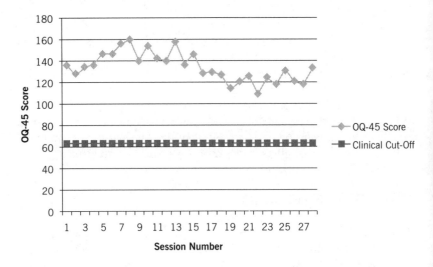

FIGURE 9.1. Assessment of Kate's progress on the OQ-45 measure.

and engage with a group of potential friends who were leading healthy lives. I hope this social support may lead to a reduction in her use of drugs, and to her feeling more affirmed by peers. The future of her current relationship will no doubt depend upon a range of factors that are beyond the scope of the current therapy that was limited by the time constraints of my University clinic. However, Kate has already developed an awareness that the only way she is going to achieve lasting change will be through developing an inner capacity to extricate herself from her current relationship and enter into more healthy, affirming relationships.

PERSONAL REFLECTIONS

The Therapist's Perspective

I found myself mesmerized by Kate's early experiences, which were so different from my own, having come from a more privileged and more intact background. During the early period of the therapy, I experienced a strong need to be the one who would rescue Kate and help her find a different trajectory. The more I experienced her childlike vulnerability and dependency, the greater my own need became to provide her with an opportunity that would foster her own sense of well-being, creativity, and vitality.

In learning about conducting long-term psychotherapy, I was also starting to learn more about myself, both as a therapist and as a person.

It was a challenge for me to acknowledge the aspects of myself of which I was becoming increasingly aware, particularly my desire to help and please others. This aspect of my personal dynamics was expressed in my work with Kate, as I was often left feeling inadequate or pressured to "do" more. I tried to keep this awareness from undermining my ability to remain present in the session and close to her feelings and experiences. However, the therapeutic journey became increasingly complex because of Kate's hospitalization and her continuing drug use.

My supervisor and I decided to seek consultation. Therapy felt like it had become stuck. Our consultant suggested that we consider several issues. First, were we expecting too much change too soon for this patient? He wondered whether therapy was really stuck, or the feeling of it reflected a countertransferential reaction. Through the consultation process, it also became clear that Kate's drug use was a serious problem. It was an addiction and also an avoidance of treatment. We talked about the use of motivational interviewing to help address Kate "where she is." Her ongoing use of drugs was surely an avoidance of her real feelings, but one that had never been openly addressed in the therapy. Our consultant also suggested that helping Kate to see her strengths, and the way these are undermined through her drug use, may be useful, as well as educating her that with her continuing use of marijuana and oxycontin it will be hard for her to understand herself more or see things differently. He suggested that the use of motivational enhancement in the context of a psychodynamically oriented, supportive experience may allow Kate to gradually extend her recognition of her "readiness for change" (Prochaska, DiClemente, & Norcross, 1992).

With the complexities surrounding her relationship with her boyfriend and her mother, Kate's relationship with me seemed to be the only one in her life that allowed her to experience (albeit transiently) a healthier sense of her self. The therapeutic relationship may provide a platform to bring things to Kate's attention, make observations about what she is doing to herself, and explore the meaning of her seemingly self-destructive behavior. It is unlikely that the therapeutic relationship alone will be sufficient for Kate to leave her partner, repair things with Mum, and enter a new healthy relationship. However, it may give her the opportunity to have one healthier relationship to help her along the way.

The Supervisor's Perspective

Gaining the perspective of an external person with insight and looking at a case anew is extremely valuable. The consultant drew attention to the degree to which both the therapist and I were avoiding the most obvious of issues before our eyes, that is, the patient's continued use of drugs, and the importance of addressing this much more directly than we had to date.

I was also able to look at the issue of the supervisee's experience in a new way. I was struck by her words, "I feel tricked, like I am the only one in the room who feels." I am aware of the degree to which the therapist was highly regarded by this patient who feels so badly about herself. I made the decision that I needed to support the therapist in better utilizing the relationship to foster optimism and realism for the patient. Following consultation, I was left with a renewed sense of hope, and perhaps a more realistic optimism, about continuing with this case.

REFERENCES

Bateman A., & Fonagy, P. (2006). *Mentalization-based treatment for borderline personality disorder: A practical guide.* Oxford, UK: Oxford University Press.

Lambert, M. J., Lunnen, K., Umphress, V., Hansen, N., & Burlingame, G. M. (1994). *Administration and scoring manual for the Outcome Questionnaire (OQ-45.1).* Salt Lake City, UT: IHC Center for Behavioral Healthcare Efficacy.

Prochaska, J. O., DiClemente, C. C., & Norcross, J. C. (1992). In search of the structure of change. In Y. Klar, J. D. Fisher, J. M. Chinsky, & A. Nadler (Eds.), *Self change: Social, psychological, and clinical perspectives* (pp. 87–114). New York: Springer.

Summers, R. F., & Barber, J. P. (2010). *Psychodynamic therapy: A guide to evidence-based practice.* New York: Guilford Press.

CHAPTER 10

THE UNCERTAIN FATHER
A Case of Low Self-Esteem

SAMUEL J. COLLIER

Aaron, a young man who struggles with feelings of competition, inferiority, uncertainty about his sexuality, and disappointment in his career, achieved significant gains in the 16-month psychotherapy described here. Initially, the therapist wisely focused on creating a good working relationship with Aaron, who was very sensitive to any hint of criticism, by consistently expressing empathy. With a strong therapeutic alliance built on this empathic stance, the therapist was able to offer comprehensive and deep interpretations that might have precipitated a major rupture in the therapeutic relationship if given too soon.

Early in the treatment, the therapist gently explored Aaron's distress about his girlfriend's flirtatiousness with other men. Building on this strong, empathic foundation, the patient began to question why he never became angry with the other men. The therapist was able to explore the transference relationship and its striking parallels with the patient's relationship with his father, and this seemed to both open up the treatment relationship and bolster the patient's confidence.

The termination, although planned, happened quickly and the patient was transferred to another therapist in the same clinic. Had the therapist had more time to work with Aaron, he might have had an opportunity to explore Aaron's feelings about termination more fully. Nevertheless, it is impressive how much insight the patient gained and how much his sense of self stabilized and strengthened in this course of treatment.

CHIEF COMPLAINT AND PRESENTATION

Aaron presented for treatment depressed and demoralized. He was an attractive, fit young man in his 30s who came across as passive and likable. His complaints centered on recurring feelings of jealousy that interfered with his romantic relationships along with uncertainty about his heterosexual identity. Aaron was analytical and inquisitive. This was his first experience with a psychiatrist or mental health professional, and he appeared genuine in his efforts to explain himself and elaborate his dilemmas. As his narrative slowly unfolded it became clear that he was often distressed and overcome by feelings of jealousy, loneliness, and inferiority. He plainly expressed a desire to understand himself better and figure out why he felt awful much of the time.

As a recent law school graduate and legal intern, Aaron struggled to stay motivated in his work. He was annoyed by his male boss who seemed to minimize his contributions and emphasized his lesser role as a legal underling. Aaron had trouble asserting himself and defending his occupational skill set. He was often assigned mundane tasks beneath his skill level but hesitated to question his boss' authority. He experienced vengeful fantasies in which he humiliated his boss in head-to-head courtroom arbitration. In reality, he avoided confrontation, and ingratiated himself and praised his boss—which left him feeling miserable and used. At times, he questioned his career choice altogether and wallowed in a feeling of weakness and career failure.

Aaron elaborated on current relational difficulties with his girlfriend. She was an attractive young professional and they had been together for several months. He felt a great sense of fulfillment at having gained her attention and engaged her in a romantic relationship. At times he indicated how lucky and unlikely he was to have ended up with such a gorgeous woman. He described in some detail how they had been acquaintances in high school, but he had never imagined having the opportunity to date her.

His involvement with her began during a chance meeting at an art event. He described experiencing a distinct confidence that day, a feeling that made him feel important and powerful. He relished the feeling and later lamented how transient it was. Aaron and his girlfriend moved in together soon after beginning to date, and their difficulties became apparent to him right away. She was vivacious and sassy but also demanding and petulant. When she focused emotional and sexual attention on him, he felt strong and empowered. When her attention drifted elsewhere, he tended to view her as nagging and unappreciative. He felt persecuted by her criticism of his procrastination and messiness. He also felt controlled by her seductive power and had difficulty interpreting subtle signs of affection. For example, he felt satisfied with physical contact but did not perceive her cooking him dinner or washing his clothes as indicators of her affection.

Aaron felt jealous and injured by his girlfriend's seemingly innate ability to attract the attention of other men. He frequently became jealous of her male peers, and tended to hyper-focus on how other men were bigger, stronger, and more suitable partners than he. Aaron described one instance when he met a particularly attractive male acquaintance of his girlfriend while out at a bar. He instantly fixated on the man's physique and obsessed over his large biceps and confident personality. Despite an appropriate introduction, he was irritated by his girlfriend's flirtatious interaction with him. At the same time, he viewed himself as submissive, undeserving, and weak, which consumed him. He felt so bad he did not even try to compete. His fixation on the competing male was so intense that he wondered whether he had homosexual feelings toward these men, especially the attractive ones with whom his girlfriend flirted. This thought was distressing, and he admitted it reluctantly.

Aaron was well aware of his jealousy and directed an immense amount of anger toward his girlfriend. His anger frequently led to verbal arguments that escalated to vicious yelling matches and threats by both parties to leave the relationship. He had difficulty controlling his temper and felt his masculinity was constantly under attack. He was aware that his girlfriend was provocative and demeaned him when threatened in the midst of an argument. Her hurtful criticism further injured him until he eventually exploded. Sometimes his outbursts evoked a submissive reaction from his girlfriend, and she would retreat from the argument and apologize. Aaron was aware that he perceived these situations in part as a victory for his masculinity but was also ashamed of his temper and fearful of being out of control.

Aaron sought refuge and support in regular attendance of Alcoholics Anonymous meetings. He had been going to meetings for years at the suggestion of his father, who was many years into sustained sobriety. Although Aaron did not have an addiction history, he described the groups as useful and comforting. There were some ebbs and flows to his attendance, but his interest reignited after fights at home or when he experienced worsening loneliness and depression. Aaron's father and girlfriend both encouraged him to maintain a connection with AA, and he responded to their requests obediently. However, there were times when he had the urge to abandon and rebel against some of the AA principles.

HISTORY

Aaron was raised in a working class urban area by his mother and father. His parents met under unusual circumstances when his father was admitted to a drug and alcohol rehabilitation program. His mother was a counselor there, and a relationship developed after his father completed the program and achieved what would be permanent sobriety from severe addiction. Aaron described his parents' meeting with some discomfort, as if he felt the romance of their relationship but could not fully embrace it.

Aaron was enamored by his father's charm, describing him as a self-made man who hustled in his climb to success as an eventual manager of a medium-sized company. He idealized his father's will, work ethic, and ability to remain optimistic. He did admit an element of grandiosity in his dad's approach to life but was fiercely loyal to him, staying in close contact over the years and often seeking his advice. Aaron seemed particularly vulnerable to ignoring some of the disappointing qualities his father had, including the history of addiction and the scandalous infidelity that later ruined his parents' marriage. He also tended to under-emphasize his success in relation to his father's despite his own high academic achievement and a healthy income. Aaron recalled a recent visit from his father when he wanted to proudly show off his new office. When his father declined the invitation, Aaron was stricken with conflict, feeling both inferior and competitive.

When Aaron first discussed his mother, he wondered if she had borderline personality disorder. He had been reading a psychology text and hypothesized about her character structure. He raised the question in an innocent and kind way, simply wondering about her self-esteem and ability to sustain healthy relationships. He told a story about how his family considered him "most like" his mother both in looks and temperament. He indicated uneasiness with this association despite expressing deep affection for her. He described how his mother was a hard worker and how she would often come home from her day job to strictly manage a meticulous household.

Aaron was uncomfortable with how critical his mother was of his father during childhood. She would often nag, criticize his father's sloppy table manners, and accuse him of being lazy and unhelpful. He felt conflicted between feeling physically and psychologically similar to his mother and feeling protective of his father's character and family loyalty.

Although the home atmosphere was intense, the family stayed together and, due to the father's occupational success, moved to an upper middle-class suburb by the time Aaron started middle school. This was a pivotal change for Aaron, who had to endure leaving his friends and integrating into a new social and economic order. In middle school, he was hypervigilant about the social hierarchy, often feeling unpopular, out of place, and undesirable. He obsessed about not being "a jock" and craved to be respected and admired. Academically, Aaron performed at an average level and found himself distracted by girls. Gaining the attention of women began to be a critical mission and also a frustration. He looked for ways to gain social status and decided to play on the baseball team.

In high school, Aaron continued his quest for popularity and admiration. He achieved social clout by joining a rock-and-roll band as a singer and for a while enjoyed significant popularity. At one point during a surge of confidence he worked up the nerve to ask out "the hottest girl" in school. He described her acceptance of him as momentous, but said he regained a sense of inferiority almost immediately after going out with her. This experience kicked off a pattern of interactions with women where he engaged when he was confident and then became progressively more insecure. This insecurity manifested as jealousy, need for admiration, and obsessive worry about inadequacy. Each relationship was tainted by his experience of feeling hurt and rejected by the previous ones. Unfortunately, his preoccupation with impending rejection led to irritability and neediness and this usually precipitated real rejection from his partners. This ultimately led to terrible loneliness and depression.

Aaron had a longer romantic relationship in high school but it eventually imploded after his jealousy and insecurity led him to mistreat his girlfriend. While feeling depressed and dejected in the ensuing months, he had a sexual experience with a group of male peers. He felt ambivalent about this and it complicated his perceptions of men and further confused him about his competitive feelings. In his description of the experience, it was clear that he felt submissive, defeated, defective, and inferior. He felt unnerved afterward and was ashamed that it had happened. There was an undercurrent of worry that his impulsive sexual behavior meant he was homosexual. He obsessed about it often, wondering if being gay was the root of his problems.

Aaron matriculated at a respectable university, pursuing interests in English and the arts. He felt invigorated by the new degree of independence and diversity of the student body, and felt a greater sense of freedom to explore artistic and social interests. He had one serious relationship in college with an attractive woman he loved. With regret, he told the story of how he excitedly initiated the relationship but was plagued by jealousy and then resented feeling controlled. Apparently, his partner tolerated the jealousy for some time, but ultimately he was desperate for more attention and impulsively cheated on her, which prompted a swift rejection.

Aaron's parents divorced after he left for college. He later learned of an affair his father had had which precipitated the separation. The father quickly moved in with his mistress and they were subsequently married. Soon after, she became pregnant with a son, his father's second. Aaron minimized the importance of this piece of family history. He expressed some ambivalence about the divorce, including relief that his father was no longer subjected to his mother's scrutiny and criticisms now that he was outside the home. Although he seemed liberated, Aaron wondered if his father should be more ashamed of the infidelity. Aaron noted that his mother was deeply affected by the family rift. He spoke about how she had "never recovered" and how his father's absence made her situation financially and emotionally tenuous. Aaron identified with his mother's pain and loneliness, and felt competing loyalties.

Following college graduation, Aaron felt indecisive about his career direction and briefly took a job working for his uncle's civil engineering firm. He admired his uncle's strength and physical resolve. The labor itself was hard but reassured him that he had power. Aaron described how the powerful feeling was slowly eroded by inferiority and competitiveness. He became preoccupied that his work peers were bigger, stronger, and more masculine. Aaron was also aware of feeling intellectually superior. He commented critically how many of the men seemed "brutish" with a limited range of interests. Over the course of several months Aaron felt progressively out of place and unwanted. When he escaped by drinking alcohol, he recalled feeling scared and "out of control." Although his drinking remained under control, Aaron worried over it and consulted his father for advice. His father encouraged him to begin a relationship with Alcoholics Anonymous (AA) and suggested that he apply to law school.

Aaron readily took his father's advice and was accepted to law school. He rationalized the decision saying that law made sense for an English major because of all the required reading and logic. His father's recommendations were clearly important but he had other competitive fantasies linked to his decision: he would become the most highly educated person in his family. The fantasy of being a powerful attorney was enticing but also uncomfortable.

Law school was challenging for Aaron. He described his academic performance as average. The competitive atmosphere was brutal and activated feelings of inferiority, which made him less assertive than others in obtaining a clerkship. Aaron criticized the aggressive attitude of his peers and longed for a less "hostile" learning environment. He felt compelled to compete but experienced significant discomfort. He rebelled by taking a casual attitude toward reading assignments and projects. Although able to graduate on time, his conflict about his academics led to difficulty obtaining a "preferred" internship following graduation. The internship he got made him feel competitive and stifled. This feeling, along with his relationship problems, pushed him to treatment.

CORE PSYCHODYNAMIC PROBLEM AND FORMULATION
Part I: Summarizing Statement

Aaron is a 31-year-old first-year attorney with chronic subclinical depression, recurrent jealousy, romantic relationship instability, and worries about inferiority. He is highly intelligent but conflicted about his stalled professional success. He complains of unhappiness, loneliness, a fleeting sense of empowerment, and anxiety about losing his girlfriend and being alone. He yearns for security and a sense of equality in his romantic and peer relationships, but often feels encroached upon, stifled, and slighted. There is a family history of addiction and dysthymia.

Part II: Description of Nondynamic Factors

Aaron falls shy of meeting diagnostic criteria for dysthymic or major depressive disorder. His father achieved sustained sobriety from a malignant addiction in his youth, and Aaron likely has a genetic vulnerability to impulsivity and substance abuse. His mother is dysthymic and obsessive. Aaron demonstrated a sensitive and passive temperament as a young child. He had adolescent onset depressive and anxiety symptoms predominately driven by his loneliness and sensitivity to rejection. There is no history of significant trauma and he had no prior psychiatric treatment.

Part III: Psychodynamic Explanation of Central Conflicts

Aaron's core psychodynamic problem is low self-esteem. His key conflict is a tendency to seek relationships that make him feel admired, strong, and powerful in order to deal with inner feelings of loneliness and rejection. He experienced early frustration with a lack of parental attunement, which bred a strong desire to be nurtured but also fueled anger about the lack of emotional nourishment. He feared losing control and succumbing to his rage. This comes out in his conflicted competitive and aggressive urges, where he wants to compete but is frightened of the outcome and instead takes a passive–submissive posture.

Aaron's fragile self-esteem is a reflection of his conflicted identification with his father and mother. His parents' unusual meeting in a drug rehab plays a central role in this identification. Aaron developed an early fear of losing control as he felt his father did in his struggle with addiction; he saw his father as inherently weak, and his participation in AA as a necessary measure to prevent relapse. During childhood, his father was so focused on regulating his dangerous urges that he was not able to adequately reassure Aaron to take risks and encourage healthy competition. He was fearful of asserting himself with his father. For example, he did not question the recommendation to attend AA despite not being an addict himself. In summary, Aaron both idealized his father and adopted a passive–submissive role to protect and stabilize his view of him as strong and stable.

Aaron's view of his mother is equally conflicted. He views her as sensitive but withholding and critical. In childhood, he resented his mother's nagging and wished for her to praise and admire his father (and him) rather than nit-pick. Her criticisms activated protective feelings as Aaron identified with his father as passive and vulnerable. However, he unconsciously worried that without his mother's tough approach his dad would succumb to temptation and start using again.

Aaron's view of his parents' relationship was further complicated by the beginning of their relationship: a boundary transgression by his counselor mother and recovering father. Aaron learned that his demanding and critical mother rescued his attractive but vulnerable father. The story of their courtship implied to Aaron that men were flawed and prone to dangerous and impulsive behavior if not kept in check. However, Aaron felt his mother was so critical and inflexible in the home environment that her behavior engendered rebellion in the form of his father's impulsive affair. In essence, being alone or in a relationship were both problematic. Without a partner, Aaron was vulnerable to making bad choices. In a relationship, he was likely to suffer criticism that would invoke impulsive anger and make him feel out of control.

Aaron recalls one instance at dinner when his mother openly criticized his father for being a sloppy eater. The more she criticized, the more the father withdrew. Aaron recalls his father distancing himself, ruminating about how his hard work was not valued, and helping less with household chores. This cycle repeated itself for many years until the marriage was compromised by his father's infidelity and ultimate departure to live with his new wife. His mother deteriorated substantially after losing her husband, becoming needy, "mushy," and dependent on Aaron for support. Consumed by her own pain, she could not fully appreciate how awful it was for Aaron to see the marriage crumble. Witnessing the failed marriage perpetuated Aaron's earlier concerns about the dangerousness of being alone and the stifling confines of being in a relationship. There was an undertone of anger at his parents for being neglectful of his feelings, but this anger was uncomfortable for him to discuss. He adapted by attempting to avoid competition, especially with his father, because of an unconscious fear that he would lose control and hurt people with his feelings or behavior.

Aaron's self-esteem difficulties were manifested in adolescence by his avid pursuit of girls and social status. He could tolerate neither being alone nor being in a relationship, and sabotaged relationships with girls by being jealous and needy. There was a constant drive to achieve social status that would soothe his concerns about being flawed and inferior. This drive caused him to become preoccupied with the "superior" qualities of other men, which was a major force driving his homosexual anxiety. For him, the homosexual impulses reflected his idealization of other powerful men and expressed his feeling inferior to them.

Aaron became intensely jealous in his current relationship after the initial satisfaction of attracting his girlfriend waned. He tried to suppress his jealousy and battled the urge to revert to a rigid gender dynamic, in which he insisted she defer to him and provide constant validation. When his girlfriend dramatically resisted his maladaptive attempts to gain her respect he would resort to either wallowing in self-pity or succumbing to angry jealousy with scathing fantasies about abandoning the relationship.

A similar manifestation of Aaron's discomfort with competition appeared in his professional environment. He wanted to feel respected in his role as a young attorney but had difficulties in his first two jobs. In his internship, he worked for a male boss who gave him menial assignments. Aaron felt insulted and deprived of the ability to prove his worth. He avoided confrontation at all costs and instead fantasized about dramatic ways to prove his superiority. Unfortunately his defensive deference did not help him achieve an improved position in the organization. His colleagues sensed his discomfort and distanced themselves, which led him to more rumination about being undervalued and manipulated.

Part IV: Predicting Responses to the Therapeutic Situation

Aaron is smart and articulate. He has a keen interest in human behavior but tends to reflect on his struggles at the expense of appreciating his impact on others. He is likely to demonstrate deference and idealization in the transference relationship, as these reactions protect him from anxiety associated with challenging the therapist more directly. He will be quite vulnerable to feeling criticized by interpretations in the treatment that mimic his mother's criticisms. His reaction to feeling criticized may include impulsive departure from treatment, which would be an obvious obstacle to therapeutic gains.

The therapist may experience a caretaking countertransference in response to Aaron's passive posture and need for admiration. While potentially useful in the early stage for alliance building, this impulse to take care of Aaron may also stall treatment gains if it leads to avoidance in making more direct interpretations out of fear of hurting Aaron's feelings. Another possible countertransference is feeling annoyed at Aaron's passivity and idealization. Showing this annoyance could interfere with his sense of safety in the therapeutic alliance.

COURSE OF TREATMENT

Aaron's treatment course was characterized by five phases: (1) building the therapeutic alliance, (2) exploring the relationship with his girlfriend, (3) understanding the impact of her pregnancy, (4) interpreting competition and caretaking in the transference, and (5) analyzing the paternal relationship and connecting it to the transference.

Building the therapeutic alliance was the initial focus of therapy. I accomplished this by empathizing with Aaron's pain, vulnerability, and anger. He was aware that he felt depressed and jealous but he could not initially connect these emotions to having a self-esteem problem. As Aaron recognized his tendency to berate himself and feel inferior he was able to explore the origin of these feelings and correct some of his distortions.

I expressed support and respect for what Aaron endured through active listening and careful clarification. Additionally, it was helpful to point out that some of Aaron's observations were realistic. For example, his girlfriend's behaviors with other men were often provocative. Successive small validations made Aaron more comfortable in treatment and he seemed to look to me as someone who took interest in him, gently challenged his distortions, and pushed for clarity about the origin of his low self-esteem.

In this first treatment phase Aaron was passive and overly deferential. There was a distinct disconnect between his professional dress and the slumped posture he assumed in the chair. Although he initially made some passing inquiries about my age and degree of experience, he tended to idealize me and look for validation and mirroring of his painful affects. I recognized Aaron's passive posture as a signal to be gentle and nurturing in the early phase of treatment. I was careful not to risk making early interpretations that would activate feelings of shame or competition and push him away from therapy.

As he became comfortable discussing his inner feelings and the therapeutic alliance consolidated, I empathized with his vulnerability. His girlfriend was a central part of the conversation and he often felt like he was in trouble, about to lose the relationship, or was fiercely indignant at her critical or withholding behavior. I sensed that our developing collaboration splinted the anxiety about examining his role in the relationship and engendered Aaron's curiosity about why his feelings were so persistent and repetitive.

Aaron described serious doubts about the sustainability of his relationship. His sense of value depended almost exclusively on his girlfriend's admiration and validation. This left him feeling vulnerable, fragile, and hypervigilant about perceived slights from her. He was annoyed, insulted, and sometimes hostile to her for a variety of reasons. The theme generally involved his discomfort with her loose boundaries with other men, or injury from her criticisms of his personal qualities, such as being messy or avoidant. It was difficult to draw his attention to this, but he tolerated it as the alliance improved. Importantly, we connected Aaron's sensitivity to criticism with an early childhood experience Aaron had with his mother.

At age 6 Aaron recalled having an accidental episode of fecal incontinence while in the grocery store. His mother had previously dismissed his requests to use the bathroom as annoying and unnecessary. Aaron remembered how his mother reacted furiously and how humiliated he felt. The experience was devastating and he associated it to earlier feelings about being a sensitive, messy boy who had difficulty maintaining self-control. He felt his mother had rigid expectations for cleanliness and order.

I pointed out that his mother had dismissed an essential bodily function and criticized him when he was unable to control himself, afterwards causing him to feel worthless, neglected, and betrayed. I suggested that his mother's inability to empathize and soothe him led to an intense desire to be understood and valued. It also engendered anxiety about feeling out of control and impulsive. Aaron was starved for attention but vigilant about real or perceived criticism, especially from women, because of early experiences of being humiliated and overwhelmed by his mother. He connected the incident in the grocery store to the present conflict with his girlfriend, and Aaron began to see that his present reactions to her criticisms were often exaggerated. He began to understand that, unlike in his childhood relationship with his mother, he had a more mature ability to communicate with his girlfriend without regressing into jealous and hostile dialogue.

Later in treatment, Aaron reported an argument with his girlfriend. They were driving to a shopping mall and had brought along lunch to save time. The couple unpacked their food in the parking lot to quickly eat before going inside to shop. Aaron was feeling confident and began joking with his girlfriend as she unwrapped a tuna fish sandwich. The joking escalated as he playfully pretended to spill the tuna on her. Aaron admitted that he had been careless and ultimately spilled tuna on her shirt. Not surprisingly she was upset and dramatically accused him of "ruining the afternoon." Aaron immediately felt intolerable shame and became angry. I clarified that he had been genuinely playful with his girlfriend and the spill was accidental. Furthermore, his girlfriend's reaction was partly justified but out of proportion to what happened. I suggested that the experience made Aaron feel humiliated and infantilized, similar to how he felt after his mother's reproaches.

However, his preoccupation with being foolish and sloppy compelled him to want his partner to keep him in check, which he later resented. I asked him why he felt he needed her to set limits on him. Aaron became annoyed with me and accused me of withholding critical advice that he needed to succeed. I suggested that he felt "out of control" and wanted me, like his girlfriend and father, to steer him away from his childish and impulsive urges. I explained that if I satisfied his request we risked infantilizing him.

Shortly after beginning treatment, Aaron reported that his girlfriend was pregnant. He was excited by this but unrealistically preoccupied with whether he was the baby's father. His paternity concerns consumed him and he could not initially appreciate other important implications of fatherhood. He expressed anxiety about whether the relationship would endure the pregnancy and that he would be left alone after the birth as his girlfriend directed her attention to the baby. He was also concerned that his girlfriend might abort the baby without his input.

I interpreted Aaron's reaction to the pregnancy as a conflict between feeling like an advocate and protector for his family and fear of inferiority and powerlessness. Aaron seemed to appreciate and understand this viewpoint and was able to tolerate significant uncertainty in the relationship, including recognition of his inability to control his girlfriend's decision about terminating the pregnancy.

Weeks later, Aaron reported that his girlfriend had decided to keep the baby. As he thought more about the pregnancy, it became clear he was developing a sense of pride and satisfaction with fatherhood. With less ambivalence he invested himself in the role of being a father. However, this stirred up an interesting conflict. On the one hand, Aaron did not want to be bound to a long-term commitment with a woman who would periodically withhold attention and provoke him. On the other hand, the idea of fatherhood was deeply satisfying and he wanted to bravely face it despite his complicated relationship struggles. His focus on being a father seemed to allow him to shift from his daily struggles with low self-esteem and instead, appreciate the essential role he would have as provider and protector. Somehow it was easier for him to tolerate his girlfriend's provocations during pregnancy, and his paternity concerns dissipated.

As the delivery neared, Aaron often reminded me that he would need to miss therapy when his girlfriend went into labor. The baby was born without complications, and he returned to treatment visibly proud with an authentic sense of satisfaction and commitment to his new responsibilities. There were residual worries that conflict with his girlfriend could lead to eventual separation. His thoughts, however, were not focused on feeling injured or rejected, but rather how to maintain a healthy bond with the baby despite potentially difficult circumstances.

Overall, fatherhood was a pivotal moment for Aaron. It helped him to look outside himself, experience less need for admiration, and focus on an altruistic purpose. I suspected that fatherhood also served other unconscious functions, such as validating his masculinity, diminishing his anxiety about homosexuality, and relaxing his more competitive urges.

As Aaron's treatment progressed, we began to explore the transference relationship more actively. The primary transference reactions were deference and idealization. Aaron had called me "Doctor" for the first several months of treatment. He tended not to attach my last name but simply said "Hi, Doctor" or "Thank you, Doctor." He was extremely polite and listened attentively when I spoke, often appearing like a pupil in a classroom. I eventually pointed out this behavior to him and he seemed surprised, as if it would be rude to act differently. I commented that, although he was certainly polite, he seemed to take particular care not to offend me. This served as an entry point to a careful discussion about competition in the transference.

Aaron wanted to see me as confident, calm, and educated. During one session, he expressed a strong curiosity to know what I was like outside of treatment. He speculated that I always felt "centered" and assumed I had a flawless relationship with a gorgeous woman. Later, he admitted to trying to find out more information about me on the Internet. I inquired about his fantasies, wondering how he would feel if his idealized assumptions proved valid or invalid. Aaron rationalized his urges to know more about me. He felt the relationship was unequal if I could withhold personal information.

I suspected Aaron had ambivalent feelings about me. Part of him wanted to completely invest his trust in me to help him feel better. On the other hand, he resented this form of dependency and preferred to compete with me for more equal footing in the relationship. Investigating my background was a risky way to express this ambivalence: discovering positive attributes about me might allow him to feel more secure and nurtured, but could also exacerbate his dependency fears, or perhaps his competitive feelings; alternatively, his investigation could ostensibly disprove some of his idealized assumptions, rendering him anxious about my competence while satisfying his urge to challenge the power differential.

At the end of one session Aaron offered to bring me coffee the following week. I noticed that his attitude seemed particularly casual that day, almost reminiscent of two friends getting together to chat. I politely declined his offer and he missed the next session. Aaron rationalized the missed appointment, but I interpreted it as a defensive reaction following my concrete reminder that our relationship was not as peers. He perceived this as a rejection and the missed appointment was his retaliation. Our discussion of his reaction was fruitful and he was interested in its meaning. After this, there were times when he arrived late that correlated with especially difficult material being discussed, but overall his attendance remained consistent.

Competition became a major treatment theme. As Aaron relayed more of his narrative I focused on this and, on one occasion, my comments precipitated a rupture in the alliance. I made an observation about Aaron's tendency to direct anger toward his girlfriend rather than at male competitors who occasionally approached her inappropriately. Over the first 7 months of treatment, I had validated the notion that his girlfriend seemed to be overly familiar with men, and now I was commenting on his role in the dynamic.

Aaron described an instance while dining with another couple when he felt the other man was being inappropriately affectionate with his girlfriend. He became envious and angry with her for allowing it and this precipitated a big argument. I pointed out that his girlfriend's behavior was not so surprising. We had discussed it extensively at that point, and Aaron's tolerance of it had improved. I then commented that he was much more likely to direct anger at her rather than the male who was intruding on his boundary. Given his prior masculinity concerns I questioned whether it would be more "manly" to directly confront a competing male than to be angry with his girlfriend. This visibly upset Aaron, who became defensive and short. He returned next session and we reexamined what happened. Aaron felt that I had been overly critical and was insinuating that he was not "manly enough" to defend his turf. He made a point of talking about how he was not afraid of fighting or pain. I conceded that my comments had a critical undertone, apologized, and empathized with how painful it was to feel criticized by someone who was supposed to be helping. Taking the time to work through Aaron's anger at me helped to reestablish the therapeutic alliance, and we launched into more discussion about his discomfort with male competition and how this manifested in the treatment.

Therapy continued to evolve, and Aaron demonstrated several more positive changes. He became bolder in the expression of his feelings without being hostile. He began to challenge my interpretations more actively, kindly pushing me to justify my assertions. He also stopped calling me "Doctor" and was increasingly poised, without pushing the boundary of being overly casual. Aaron said he felt much better and more optimistic about his future. He had worked hard to react less to his girlfriend's histrionic behavior and push for more responsibility at work. He expressed one final therapeutic goal, which was to discuss his father. At the same time, he asked to reduce his treatment frequency from weekly to biweekly. I initially agreed, wanting to respect his autonomy and independence, but later changed my mind, as I suspected his request to reduce frequency stemmed from his discomfort about exploring competitive feelings he had about his father.

At his next appointment, I brought up my concerns, interpreting his request to come less often as a way to avoid competing with me. I hypothesized that Aaron's growing assertiveness felt dangerous and he worried that challenging me more directly, as he had been, would lead to rejection. Aaron quickly agreed to resume weekly sessions, rationalizing the decision by saying he wanted to learn more about his family dynamics. In the next session, however, he was distressed. He told me he was "worried about being messed up." He felt my suggestion to stay with weekly treatment meant that he was flawed and weak. He was ashamed that he had not argued with me more and had later resented being "told what to do." I suggested that his reaction had a temporal relationship with our decision to address his relationship with his father, and suggested we proceed.

As we resumed weekly sessions I empathized with Aaron's anger and clarified that he had avoided being more directly angry at me fearing he would lose control and risk hurting me. Aaron described a parallel anxiety in his paternal relationship. His father had recently been forced to leave his long-standing job and take a new position selling office equipment. During a recent visit, Aaron had had lunch with his dad, who chatted eagerly about equipment sales and his marketing strategy. Aaron found himself bored and annoyed with the conversation and how it was exclusively focused on his father. I asked him why it was so difficult to communicate his annoyance and talk more about himself. Aaron responded by describing a deep-seated fear of confronting his father. He admitted that he was not impressed by his father's new job, and he worried that somehow if he expressed his concerns more directly this would destabilize his father and potentially make him prone to relapsing back into drug use. We clarified together a similar transference fear of losing control and damaging our relationship. Aaron worried that challenging me too much might have grave consequences and I connected this anxiety to his desire to come to session less frequently.

TERMINATION

The decision to terminate came somewhat artificially, as I was completing my residency and planning to take a job out of state. I had delayed broaching the topic until about 8 weeks prior to my move date. I was aware of my resistance to terminating the treatment because it had been satisfying and successful but far from complete. I felt guilty about abandoning Aaron and felt he had made great strides to feel more secure and confident by way of tolerating many unpleasant feelings and staying the course in our relationship. It seemed cruel to leave him when we had achieved such a steady therapeutic rhythm.

Aaron received the news of impending termination with some surprise. He expressed disappointment but also gratitude for the relationship we had developed. He inquired about where I was going, what role I would have, and if it was possible for him to continue with me. I disclosed my decision to accept an academic job out of state. "You mean you'll be a professor?" Aaron said with genuine warmth and excitement. I commented that it seemed important for him to have an internal image of me being successful. He responded by stating his intentions to continue therapy and asking for my help with choosing a new therapist. I suspected the quick shift of focus to finding a new therapist was defensive and helped him cope with the relationship loss. I had already planned for a transfer and discussed with him the various options. Ultimately, he chose to continue treatment with a colleague in the same clinic.

ASSESSMENT OF PROGRESS

Aaron made significant progress in treatment over a period of 16 months. He understood and tolerated his repeating painful feelings of jealousy, fear of loneliness, vulnerability, and losing control. He was able to clarify many of his underlying relationship wishes including the need for closeness, admiration, and respect.

He made significant changes in how he managed his romantic relationship, demonstrated an enhanced ability to tolerate criticism from his girlfriend, and began to understand that he did not have to oscillate between soliciting emotional closeness and tolerating her bossy provocations. Aaron slowly integrated a more realistic view of himself and his girlfriend. He began to see that he had strengths and a stable set of personal virtues mixed with vulnerabilities derived from an early lack of nurturing. The more he tolerated emotional volatility at home, the more respect he gained from his girlfriend and this increased his sense of stability.

Aaron's concept of masculinity changed substantially as well. In the beginning, he maintained a rigid view that men should be admired, nurtured, and unchallenged by their partners. He was strictly wed to this view of himself but initially unclear about how it had developed. The psychotherapy clarified that his rigid view of masculinity was an unconscious way to deal with his early experience of deprivation and desire for emotional attunement. Aaron also stopped worrying that he was gay, which was a source of great upset at the beginning of treatment. Although Aaron's psychosexual development revealed an obvious pattern of heterosexual arousal, he was frequently distressed by his past homosexual feelings. He seemed to latch on to the idea that "you're gay or you're not" with a rigidity similar to his initial concept of masculinity. Clarifying that his homosexual feelings related to his feeling of inferiority and struggle with competition increased his confidence in his sexuality and his sexual relationship.

Lastly, Aaron gained some insight into his tendency to avoid competition with other men. This had delayed his ascent in the ranks in his law firm and, in turn, increased his sense of inferiority. As attention was paid to disappointments in his relationship with his father, and his fears about hurting his father, he realized that healthy assertiveness was nontoxic and advantageous, rather than harmful.

As the treatment came to a close, Aaron still faced many difficulties. His girlfriend's behavior had not changed, which meant that he had to tolerate ongoing provocation and was vulnerable to angry regressions. He still fought with her, and near the end of treatment there was serious doubt about whether they would remain together, despite being parents of a young infant girl. While still prone to injury from insults and arguments, Aaron clearly had more insight into his dynamics. Treatment helped him realize that he had value and skills that were not contingent on her reactive character assessments. When he regressed he knew why. The thought of being alone was not as terrifying as it had been previously, and he tolerated the uncertainty of his relationship and how he might be forced to handle being a single father.

This was Aaron's first treatment experience and he approached it with curiosity and open mindedness. His initial treatment goals were quite sensible, and focused on feeling less jealous, angry, and worried about his sexuality. As treatment continued, his goals expanded to include achieving a richer understanding of his early family experience and ambivalence about his attachment figures. Overall, Aaron was satisfied with his progress over 16 months. He was realistic about expecting slow but meaningful change.

CHAPTER 11

THE REAL ELMER FUDD

A Case of Low Self-Esteem

C. PACE DUCKETT

Matt, the insecure young man depicted in this case, tried to live out a typical male fantasy of money, girls, and sports cars, only to find that he felt lonely and anxious. The case history describes a distinct presenting problem, a nicely developing engagement with the therapist, increasing insight with new, more accurate perceptions of others, and finally, real behavioral change. The arc of this successful psychotherapy demonstrates a classical coherence that is rare, as treatments are rarely so clear and well-characterized.

The therapist recognized a powerful ongoing positive transference that is both an expression of the patient's problem and a therapeutic experience in its own right. There are a couple of rather dramatic moments in the patient's life in which his sensitivity to rejection becomes so apparent that he cannot escape it. In the second of these incidents, enough work had already been accomplished in therapy that he was able to behave quite differently from his usual pattern, and this new experience further consolidated his therapeutic gains.

CHIEF COMPLAINT AND PRESENTATION

As the crisp fall air set in to Manhattan, Matt found himself walking absent-mindedly down the bustling New York streets. He had only been there for 2 weeks when he abruptly ran into Amber, his ex-girlfriend. The interaction was brisk, short, and awkward. Upon separating, Matt felt a pit of nothingness and despair. The following day at his new job with a small record label, thoughts began to swirl in his mind. He removed himself quietly from the office and went out on the street corner to get some air. But with all the people passing furiously around him, his mind continued to churn. Dwarfed by the buildings, he felt Manhattan was swallowing him. He imagined he saw Amber around every corner. Was he going to bump into her? The spinning turned to dizziness, and the dizziness into . . . collapse. He was not aware that anyone had called 911, and he barely remembered the EMS ride to the ER. But once there, the doctors told him he might have had a seizure; apparently he had had some twitching and confusion while on the ground. The EEG and ECG were all within normal limits, but he ended up on a prescription for an antiepileptic nevertheless.

Many months later a similar episode happened. Alone, recently unemployed, and basically hiding out in his apartment, he found himself scared about the rising pressure in his chest. With no one to call, and without health insurance, he took a cab to the nearest emergency room. But rather than going in, he sat outside, pinned against a brick wall, his heart racing, short of breath, "thoughts going all crazy." He comforted himself by saying, "If it is a heart attack, at least I'm close to help." Several hours passed before Matt eventually calmed down and found his way back to his apartment. Later that night he decided he needed to go home—to his parent's home, that is. It was at this point that he also decided to seek help for his depression and anxiety.

When Matt first strolled into the office he was wearing what would later become his trademark fashion statement: a stiff brimmed black baseball cap with the boldly branded insignia "*Alife*." I amused myself trying to phonetically pronounce the label staring back at me: "Alive" or was it "A life"? Momentarily frustrated, I refocused on the young man in front of me. He told me he was planning to move out of New York City and back to his parents' suburban home in New Jersey, and he couldn't commit to any further sessions until he had actually made the transition. He just wanted to find a therapist before he moved back to work through "some issues."

HISTORY

Matt was 26 years old and had grown up in southern New Jersey. He was the only child of a Caucasian mother and an Asian father. His grandfather was an American GI who fathered a child with a local woman while stationed abroad in Asia. The biracial progeny of this relationship, Matt's father, was apparently rejected by both parents and raised by a surrogate "godmother." Matt alluded to his own confusion over the identity of his father's biological mother. Matt's mother was a child of the

60s from a straight-laced, "by-the-book" suburban family. Despite her proper upbringing, Matt's mother eloped while away in Korea on a Peace Corps mission without telling her parents. He described his mother as an organized, competent, and intelligent woman with a high-level managerial position in academia. She was not only bright, but also protective and nurturing. He confessed that she was perhaps "too good of a mother, sometimes." And he admitted that she made things so easy for him that he sometimes doubted whether he could survive on his own. Matt described his mother as the primary caretaker and provider for the household.

He noted disdainfully that his father had not worked for the previous 8 years and had become increasingly withdrawn and dysfunctional. Matt recognized that one of his "biggest issues" was with his dad. Seeing his father sit on the couch day after day talking about how lonely the dog would be if he were not there to give it company was excruciating. Matt occasionally lamented, "I wish this person did something. I mean, why hasn't he done his own thing?"

But these frustrations were hard for Matt to express given the actual fragility of his father's emotional and cognitive condition. The parallels between his father's dysfunction and his own stagnation remained unexpressed and were easily projected out onto his father's inadequacies. Matt conceded his father could barely communicate, and said talking with him "was like having the same conversations over and over again." He feared there might be something deeply wrong with his father. (It was only later in treatment that his family sought out a neurologic workup that definitively diagnosed his father with Alzheimer's dementia.)

Matt's own childhood diagnosis of juvenile rheumatoid arthritis had left him with bouts of pain episodes throughout his youth. As he got older, he continued to fear their onset, but he also became self-conscious of how others perceived his functional limitations.

While identifying strongly with his Asian side, Matt was embarrassed that he was not bilingual. He had spent a number of years living in Asia and going to school there between the ages of 9 and 13. He admitted this was a lonely period, knowing only two other American kids abroad at the time. Upon returning to the states for middle school, Matt felt the intensity of being an outsider. He predominantly befriended the social outcasts and remembered, painfully, the accusations of being "a poser" when he dressed in skater clothes at the local park. However, this rejection and suspicion by the other boys was confusingly compounded by the attention he began to receive from the girls, who were attracted by his exotic looks. But what he didn't see was the boys' resultant jealousy of this outsider. Strained relationships with men continued through much of his early years, despite Matt's efforts to be "super cool" and generous to his friends.

Matt's college years continued some of these trends. Women apparently found his tall, dark, and mysteriously handsome leading man looks hard to resist. He fell easily into a fast crowd. Drugs, clubs, and jetsetter road trips escalated, with mom just paying off the credit card bill as it came due. With "a hottie" on his arm and a bunch of friends to hang with he finally felt he had arrived. But that outsider feeling, that question of being a "poser," lingered below the surface. On graduating from college, Matt was presented with a surprise. His recently deceased maternal grandfather, the by-the-book suburban one, had left him a trust fund amounting to $700,000!

His post college years in LA and Manhattan were cloaked in the newest styles, the most bohemian apartments, and best of all, his prized two-door Mercedes Benz CLS convertible. His first serious girlfriend in LA was a gorgeous, strong, and ambitious young woman named Amber. He was smitten. Life seemed good.

The relationship advanced rapidly and with an almost dependent level of intensity. Matt always felt compelled to be available whenever she wanted. And whatever she wanted he felt compelled to give. The clubs and restaurants were always the trendsetting spots. Buying rounds for his west coast posse just seemed like a stand-up thing to do. Pulling up in the sports car to hand the keys to the valet and escort his lady to the reserved table made Matt feel like "the man." However, when the sun rose, and his girlfriend left for work, he was alone. Anxiety always seemed to creep up in the morning. It was a paralyzing, "can't get out of bed," type of anxiety.

Matt knew he needed something to do with his life. A short unpaid internship at a skateboard factory left him feeling unsatisfied and not particularly appreciated. As the relationship with Amber progressed, his doting turned to jealous suspicion. His accusations frequently led to tension and arguing. Matt preferred to whisk her away to some island adventure for a fortnight to do nothing. But, upon returning, as she went back to work, he would find himself on the couch, absorbed in self-loathing insecurity. The time seemed to be flying by, about as fast as his brokerage account was dwindling. But despite this frozen panic, Matt's response was to focus on what more he could do for Amber. How could he keep *her* happy? Months drifted during what Matt described as a long extended breakup. Things ended in a vague way, with her moving to New York City to pursue a career in fashion.

Stranded, alone, plastered to an expensive black leather sofa, Matt felt depression sink in. The self-loathing he experienced led to intense feelings of guilt and worthlessness. The previously paralyzing anxiety progressed to overt neurovegetative symptoms of depression. In session he described frequent bouts of crying, "Why doesn't anybody want to be around me, why doesn't anyone ever call?" Questions of his adequacy penetrated the stillness of the night.

Matt's relationships with his male friends suffered as well. He realized some of his tenuous ties had been maintained mostly because of his girlfriend. Without her, these "friends" seemed more like recipients of his misguided and self-absorbed philanthropy. Rounds of drinks and rides in the Benz engendered more feelings of "who does this dude think he is" rather than a genuine connection of gratitude. Matt struggled with why his super-nice-guy demeanor began to be treated disrespectfully. One day, an aggressively tense argument with his roommate left him almost paranoid and cowering in his room. During the incident, his roommate's heated accusation that "no one ever liked you anyway, Roberts" seared its way onto his memory. Perhaps it was true, he feared.

Months passed in southern California. Matt consulted a few "Hollywood docs" who prescribed "whatever pills I wanted." While a couple of trials of benzodiazepines took the edge off the anxiety, it was the calming effect of Percocet that eased the pain and suffering. He justified his blissfully numbing opiate dependency by attributing it to the real arthritic pain that crippled him daily. His juvenile rheumatoid arthritis had waxed and waned over the years. But connecting this worsening pain to his depression and anxiety was something he remained unaware of. He started to feel trapped inside his apartment and viewed the West Coast as part of his problem. Furthermore, he longed to work things out with Amber. So he made plans to move to New York City; perhaps he could prove his worth to Amber just by following her there.

CORE PSYCHODYNAMIC PROBLEM AND FORMULATION

Part I: Summarizing Statement

Matt was a 26-year-old male who presented to therapy with anxiety and mild depressive symptoms that were punctuated by occasional panic attacks. He described feelings of inadequacy, worry, self-doubt, and a strong need for reassurance in his intimate relationships. He sought help after a distant romantic breakup and his subsequent relocation home left him feeling very alone. Matt wasted several years after college without finding a clearly defined occupational path.

Part II: Description of Nondynamic Factors

At the time of presentation, Matt did not meet criteria for a major depressive disorder, but clinical history was indicative of full episodes in the past. His low-level mood symptoms were prominently pervaded by worry and insecurity. His father had a childhood history of neglect and subsequent depression in his adulthood. There was strong evidence of his father's deteriorating cognitive condition, but this was undiagnosed at the time Matt initiated treatment. His medical history revealed juvenile rheumatoid arthritis (JRA) that led Matt to experience chronic fluctuating bouts of pain throughout his life.

Part III: Psychodynamic Explanation of Core Conflicts

Matt's core psychodynamic problem is low self-esteem. The main conflicts involve early feelings of being different and defective and a defensive need to hide his feared inadequacies through an overt grandiosity.

Matt's early diagnosis of JRA at age 1½ and subsequent bouts of frequent pain contributed to an experience of self that felt damaged. As a child he rarely let anyone know that he had JRA, embarrassed that they might ridicule him. Adulthood flareups of pain would lead to shame, withdrawal, and an overall sense of helplessness. Explanations to bosses about his physical limitations made him feel judged, as if he were only making excuses about his work performance. Medical management was frequently experienced by Matt as neediness, and only made him feel desperate, misunderstood, and weak. When he complained incessantly about the chronic pain to loved ones, this would inevitably exhaust their sympathy and leave Matt feeling rejected and alone. Alternately, hiding his pain and treatments would leave him feeling damaged and alienated.

Matt's relationship with his parents contributed to feelings of low self-esteem. His father's psychological frailty resulted from a rejected and neglected childhood as the unwanted progeny of wartime strife. Matt's identification with his father was particularly difficult during his father's cognitive decline, which coincided with Matt's own occupational stagnation and the exhaustion of his trust fund. His identification with his father's deficits led to feeling fearful he would become like his father. Matt's subsequent anger at his father triggered guilt and feelings of being unworthy.

His relationship with his mother was particularly close and communication was frequent. Matt postulated that his mother felt guilty about the pain he experienced from his early diagnosis of JRA. She accommodated any distress or suffering he felt, and met all of his needs. Matt was not only excused from household chores and basic responsibilities, but even the distress of not having the latest video game was alleviated by always giving in to his demands. His mother's overcompensation throughout Matt's childhood had contributed to his feeling helpless and needy.

Matt's peer relationships during his latency years were riddled with perceived rejection. Transitions abroad and subsequently relocations back to the United States always left him feeling like a foreigner in a land he was supposed to call home. His exotic looks and questions concerning identity emphasized his feelings of difference. He experienced playground taunts of being a "poser" and not part of the gang as rejections that only served to reinforce his feared inadequacies. Thus, his defensively adopted alt-bad-boy-outsider image just led to further social marginalization.

Matt's biracial identity, culture, and ethnicity were an important topic in the therapy. His ambivalent feelings toward his Asian father were reflected in his love for the traditional cuisine of this father's homeland and his shame and regret over his lack of knowledge of other customs. He felt like a failure in his inability to become proficient in his father's tongue and saw his father's insistence that they speak English at home as an expression of his father's mixed feelings about his own background. Indeed, forming a more holistic and inclusive bicultural identity with real meaning became one of Matt's goals.

In late adolescence, his masculine good looks received the admiring attention of the opposite sex. But relationships were often intense, fawning, and dependent as Matt desperately sought reassurance to counter his low self-esteem. Jealous behaviors and an endless focus on pleasing inevitably led to tension. The eventual breakups were routinely experienced as dejection and further proof of his true inadequacy. With male friends, his self-consciousness led him to overcompensate in ways that came off as inauthentic, or even arrogant at times. His large trust fund was mostly used to buttress his fragile sense of self. But the reality was that it distanced him from his peers, delayed any occupational pursuits, and made him feel fake. He began to feel the hollowness of his materialistic preoccupations. The sports car, designer clothes, and women only reinforced the reality of his squandered inheritance, and rather than representing his success, they became paradoxical symbols of his own lack of achievement.

Matt did show a number of strengths that will aid him in his therapeutic work, including curiosity about himself, perseverance, and an ability to express his feelings.

Part IV: Predicting Responses to the Therapeutic Situation

However, Matt's motivation for change will conflict with the negative paternal transference he may develop toward the therapist. Transference issues of idealization and competition will likely lead to countertransference feelings of grandiosity or rescue fantasies for the therapist. Overall, the goals of treatment were to help Matt develop a more realistic and positive image of himself and to become less vulnerable to feelings of rejection in his relationships.

COURSE OF TREATMENT

Therapy began with an exploration of Matt's negative fantasies about himself and sought to create a link between major life events and his current difficulties. A newly constructed narrative looked at the origins of these fantasies and began to connect them to patterns in his current relationships that led to feelings of rejection and inadequacy. The middle phase of treatment looked at his own distorted perceptions of himself and how he misperceived how others were treating him. This new understanding allowed for a nonjudgmental context to understand how his life happened the way it did. The overall plan was to make links to the defensive structures he erected as a protective shield against feeling vulnerable and inferior, and to focus on what changes could be made and what could not. During these explorations, I paid particular attention to any ruptures in empathy within the therapeutic relationship. These would have been exemplified by Matt feeling misunderstood or rejected and possibly acted out by any cancellations or no shows.

Once Matt had officially moved back to his parents' home, and back into his childhood room, therapy started. He seemed motivated, engaged, but also very needy at first. He chose a time slot in the weekly schedule that was early in the morning, citing his need for something, anything, to get him out of bed. This became the topic of many of our early sessions. It was not long after opening his eyes in bed that a flood of panic would render him motionless. He dreaded the mornings, not only because *he* had nothing to do, but because "the person" downstairs had nothing to do either. The notion of joining his father on the couch in front of the TV infuriated him. Matt frequently complained, "Why doesn't he do anything . . . he just sits there all day long watching TV. I can't even have a real conversation with him. It's just the same thing over and over and over again. It's either about the weather or the dog. I mean, who cares about the damn dog. It's a dog. That's all. If my mom and I say we want to do something, my dad says, 'But what about the dog, we can't leave the dog at home, she'd miss us'."

The first phase of therapy was focused on creating a link between the origins of Matt's low self-esteem and how this self experience was expressed in his daily relationships. It was also the beginning process of developing a new narrative of his life. Whenever Matt would get into these frustrated and angry rants about his father's couch sitting he used a certain voice to mimic his father. It sounded like a drunk Elmer Fudd searching for a "Waskelly wabbit. . . . Uhh where did he go. . . . Uhh where did he go?" There was a loathsome condescension in his voice. Usually these rants were followed by guilt-ridden expressions of sympathy toward his father.

Matt admitted his underlying worry about what was actually going on with his father. He just was not the same anymore. Something medically or psychologically was really wrong. By the description of his father's memory and communication difficulties, I thought Matt was probably right. It was hard for him to see his father so defeated, it angered him, it scared him, and it caused panic every morning. It was not difficult to empathize with Matt about how hard it must be to wake up and walk down the stairs to join his father on that couch.

I spent the first couple of months of treatment supporting Matt, reassuring him, and giving him practical advice. Matt started on a selective serotonin reuptake inhibitor; we titrated the dose up slowly while discontinuing the antiepileptic medication. Sessions began with a palpable panic-stricken anxiety about what he was going to do that day and ended with a sense of calm optimism. He seemed to find hope in himself, as long as someone else believed he could do it. Matt lamented his lack of male role models and openly longed for "a normal dad"—someone who could give him some career advice, or help him with his finances, or even just talk about girls. The transference aspect of this was readily evident when he sought reassurance. He became reflective when I interpreted that his longing for my positive regard was related to his wish for a stronger relationship with a stronger father.

Aside from his insecurities, Matt was actually quite warm and funny, even self-effacing at times. Laughter was common and comfortable. But so were silences. Matt felt more and more like he could trust me. I began to clarify and explore his feeling of insecurity. "You seem worried that others will view living at home as inadequate, or just not cool for a 26-year-old." Or "You're anxious that not having a job right now is an indication that you're not capable of succeeding." These comments were acceptable to him because of the alliance that had been previously established.

As Matt became comfortable with his old stomping ground he realized he did have friends. Not guys who had been "friended" through the glitzy party scene, just good old-fashioned high school buddies. He began getting out of his parents' house more often, running errands and hanging out. He realized he was not trying to impress anyone here, as he had been in New York and LA. Nevertheless, Matt was critical of one friend in particular. Tom sat around drinking beer and watching TV, and in sessions Matt mocked him, using that same Elmer Fudd voice. But when his friend got a job cooking in a local restaurant, Matt appeared down and frustrated. He initially complained that that type of job was below him and he could do better. We discussed his jealousy of Tom's actually having a job while Matt still struggled to find anything.

This comparison reinforced Matt's feeling of inadequacy in comparison to a peer he thought himself superior to. Once, when he was describing how inadequate he felt while couchbound in LA, he used his Elmer Fudd to criticize himself. It was almost verbatim in content and tone to the mocking of his father. Matt proceeded to describe that time period, but when Elmer Fudd's defeated tone resurfaced, I brought it to Matt's attention. He acknowledged it, but seemed resistant to explore its meaning.

Over the following weeks I continued to connect any description of his father with his own frustrations of himself. I used a particular Elmer Fudd moment to summarize the meaning of this. While Matt wished to be perceived as successful and popular he had underlying fears about his adequacy as an adult man. These anxieties were not only stoked whenever he confronted his father's declining functioning, but were exacerbated by his own frustrating lack of progress. Matt was not just afraid of the similarities with his father, he was fearful that he *was* his father. And this caused paralysis.

Being back in his old neighborhood offered some unexpected opportunities. He picked up a conversation with Chad, a neighbor he had not known well. Chad was on the young side, married, with school-age kids. He was a businessman, an entrepreneur who had recently sold a startup company and was developing some new ideas. Coolest of all, to Matt: this guy loved cars. One of Chad's business ideas was for a string of carwashes and detailing shops catering to high-end automobiles. Matt talked shop and fed off the shared passion with Chad. Matt expressed an interest in developing a marketing plan for expanding the existing shop, and began to work for Chad.

The crippling morning anxiety began to decrease, and Matt seemed excited about business and entrepreneurship. It did not hurt the excitement when Chad showed him his Lamborghini in the garage. Matt's tasks were basic. He detailed cars and cleaned the shop. On rainy days he canvassed community businesses with flyers and spoke with people. Receiving his first paycheck felt good, and his mood was clearly improving. He found an apartment in the city and moved out of his parents' house. He had promised himself, "job first, then apartment," the independence strengthening him.

The second stage of therapy focused on working through Matt's current relationship patterns. We sought to identify his defensive style and how behavior repeated in predictable and understandable ways. It was around this time that Matt met the younger sister of an old college friend. Alejandra was a Brazilian beauty who was finishing her final year in pharmacy school. She was bright, smart, and full of energy; the two of them hit it off immediately even though Matt wondered about her maturity level. The relationship picked up quickly as Matt began to devote his attention to her. He liked the way he felt around her, big and strong in comparison to her petite frame. He liked the way she looked up to his age and experience. When she looked at him, he felt like a man.

But as the weeks passed, the initial glow began to be replaced by pangs of insecurity, fear, and even jealousy. Why didn't she initiate contact? Why was he always texting her first, always going to her place? Maybe she wasn't that into him? What was wrong with him? Was she cheating on him? Why hasn't she updated her Facebook status? There was a cycle. Matt got anxious about each delayed text message. He expressed his helplessness by asking for more support and reassurance at each session. However, by his description of their time together, it was evident that Alejandra was interested in him and even excited about their new relationship. We slowly began to work through the seeming discrepancy between his fears and the reality of their relationship.

The cycles could be vicious and frequent. A typical pattern might start when Alejandra was busy with personal obligations. He would become worried and try to confirm that her plans were innocuous, often through asking suspicious questions and sending serial texts. This jealous and anxiety-driven behavior eventually consumed him with guilt and self-reproach. He would then spend the next few days doting on her and being at her beck and call. He felt terrible about himself when she was not with him and increasingly needed her appreciation and attention to feel worthy.

One evening, Alejandra reminded Matt that she had her annual meeting with her academic advisor. The pharmacy professor had offered to take Alejandra to a congratulatory dinner to discuss career paths and long-term plans. But as she got ready for her dinner and walked out of the bedroom, Matt's temper began to simmer. "How do I look?" she asked. "Fine, I guess," Matt replied, as he looked her black dress up and down and noted the amount of makeup she wore. "What is this, a school thing or a date?" She brushed off his question, nervous about meeting her mentor on time and paused before rushing out the door. "I'll probably be done around 9:30 if you want to meet up with me afterwards," she said, reassuringly kissing him goodbye on the couch. So there he sat, alone. Minutes felt like forever. He couldn't stop thinking about who this advisor was. Why had he not heard more about him? Was he young or old? "I'll bet he's young and sleazy and likes to take out these undergrad girls," he thought. Once 9:00 hit, Matt sent his first text, "u almost done?" No reply. Panic built as 9:30 came. She should be finished. Still no response, where was she? Had she lied to him? Obsessions swirled and slowly the text messages started to fly: "are u finishd yet?" "why aren't u responding?" "where are u?"

By 10:00 Matt was pacing in front of the couch. He could not stand it any longer. He had to check on her. When he brusquely walked into the restaurant and found them in the dining area, the glare he received from Alejandra was chilling. He sheepishly introduced himself to her advisor and explained "I just wasn't sure when you'd be finished." The professor was polite and professional and after settling the bill left the couple together in what must have been a very awkward silence.

When Matt described the embarrassment, he barely hid his self-criticism. He was convinced he had permanently messed everything up. Alejandra must barely be able to stand what a loser he is. He berated himself. He felt she did not meet his profuse apologies with much understanding. Was she done with him? Matt's mood plummeted during episodes like this. I asked him, "What do you think you were feeling that led to going to the restaurant?" I continued with, "If your worst fears had come true, how do you think this would have made you feel?" And I explored what he thought his girlfriend was reacting so negatively to.

Matt's reflections on his own fear of inadequacy allowed us to focus on the pattern that kept repeating itself. I explained that there seemed to be a lot of insecurity he had about the relationship, especially his worry that he was not attractive and appealing enough to keep Alejandra's interest. He would project these insecurities onto specific situations and make her into an unfaithful, untrustworthy girlfriend. This projection only served to exacerbate his anxiety, especially when he was alone with nothing to do. In order to manage his discomfort he felt compelled to reassure himself of her affection with rather intrusive behavior. The behavior had become almost compulsive in its quality. And the end result was an irritated, angry, distancing girlfriend who felt smothered. Finally, he ended up feeling worthless, with his original fears of inadequacy being reinforced.

At first Matt sought reassurance that his feelings of inadequacy were only internal and not reality. During times of heightened anxiety, it helped to offer this reassurance, saying, "Matt, there's nothing actually inherently wrong with you, you're fine, you're basically 'good enough' which is okay . . . you just *fear* that you aren't . . . and this fear makes you act in ways that aren't helpful." He was able to come up with some more appropriate behaviors when he began to feel anxious and was tempted to snoop or ask too many questions. He finally concluded, "I just need to chill."

Through our work together Matt realized that he frequently focused on outward things to make him feel good, such as female affection, material items, and even his therapist's approval. While transference was not a major focus of the treatment and was rarely interpreted directly, this was a moment when I pointed out his need for positive affirmation and his fear of critical judgment. "When you find yourself feeling anxious or helpless, I notice that you increasingly look outside yourself to feel okay."

In the next phase of therapy we worked much more explicitly on his behavior in this cycle of insecurity and defense. Matt described an incident when he and Alejandra were at a bar and ran into some Brazilian acquaintances. Alejandra launched into fluent Portuguese while Matt helplessly watched these men talk to his girlfriend. He boiled when they flirtatiously touched her arm and brushed her hair, all the time laughing. Matt hated South American men who exuded sexual confidence and machismo. He had momentary fantasies of punching them in their face and tearing them apart. But mostly he sulked in the dark corners of the bar the rest of the night.

We discussed Matt's aggressive competitiveness with men and how it went with his sense of inadequacy. We were also able to identify his obsequious and genial attitude toward the LA crew as a reaction formation. Matt's laying down his platinum card for rounds of drinks could more easily be understood as competition, rather than just a cool gesture from a friend. He reflected on his former roommates' comment, "No one ever liked you anyway, Roberts," and saw that his competitiveness was evident to others and not very conducive to friendship.

Matt still fought back the urge to check up on Alejandra. Though he felt ashamed of doing it, he checked her text messages and call logs when she left her phone unattended. He came in one day and admitted that he had found something and did not know what to do. It really concerned him. He hesitantly described the text message. It was an image "of some dude's penis." He tried to reassure himself that she had not even responded to the text and there did not appear to be much contact between them. The message was months old. But why did she still keep it saved? Could she be cheating on him? He didn't think so. Who was the picture of? We discussed his fears of infidelity, but also his acknowledgment that things had been going rather well between them recently. She had been sleeping over almost every night and had practically moved her stuff into his apartment. I shifted the exploration away from his fears of her cheating and onto how the image made *him* feel. He seemed to get quieter and almost shrunk into the couch. I asked him directly, "What is it that bothers you most about this image, if you're not really worried that she's cheating on you?" He was slow to answer, but eventually said, "The picture is not just some dick, it's a really big dick." He paused and I left some silence. "I mean, I've always felt, you know, average, or at least big enough, but not compared to this. If this is what she wants, I mean why does she still have it saved on her cell phone?"

I acknowledged that of course it was hard for him to have seen that image and that it did not seem to make him feel very good about himself. I realized that despite Matt being 6' 2" and built like a rugby player, he actually felt small. We were able to explore the meaning of the image in terms of his sense of adequacy as a male. He appeared to relax and become more comfortable.

He decided not to confront Alejandra about the image and instead, "just chill." He also admitted that snooping in her cell phone only increased his worries, and he was going to stop. As it happened, a few months later, Alejandra actually mentioned to Matt that some guy she and her friend had met months ago sent her a sleazy picture of his penis. She laughingly said, "I just don't get guys, do they really think we're gonna like that. At least you have class, Matt, and you'd never do something like that." Matt smiled to himself glad he had never brought it up. Perhaps he was the bigger man.

One day he brought up some concerns he had with the antidepressant he had been taking and suggested that he might be having side effects. Matt said, "I think I'm having sexual side effects, Zoloft causes that, doesn't it?" He admitted that sometimes he had trouble sustaining an erection and occasionally could not reach orgasm. I empathized and confirmed that these were indeed side effects that could be caused by the SSRI medications. But as the session went on he continued to describe the immense distress this caused him. He felt particular pressure coming from Alejandra. If he could not orgasm, she questioned whether she no longer "did it for him"? Was he still attracted to her? This made Matt feel anxious about his performance. Sometimes he got panicked before sex fearing that he could not sustain and that she would be displeased.

As I explored this intimate territory, Matt slowly explained they had sex multiple times per day. He was not bragging, and he was genuinely distressed that his performance and potency were inadequate. This feeling led him to feel compelled to satisfy her, but fearful that if he did not finish she would get upset. When she was upset, he felt strongly that he needed to do more to please her. It was clear that Alejandra was rather insecure herself and this first serious sexual relationship resulted in her own neediness to feel attractive. I commented that it sounded like he was functioning normally the first few times he had sex, but that by the fourth or fifth, he must just be exhausted.

We explored why it was so difficult to just let her know that he was fine, that he actually was satisfied. He began to see the dynamic of mutual insecurity and was able to talk through what he might say to her to alleviate the pressure he felt without making her feel rejected. We were able to talk about his focus on the SSRI and his need for something external to be causing the unsustainable sex. Their relationship seemed to be strengthened over the next few months by his increased insight, comfort with himself, and ability to communicate with his girlfriend.

A sense of trust developed as our sessions continued. Matt seemed willing to confront issues more introspectively, and he seemed comfortable talking about most everything. He shared the difficult experience of his father's diagnosis with Alzheimer's disease, tearing up as the immensity of this loss sank in. He knew this day was coming, and seemed prepared for the shifting roles. Matt began to allow himself to focus on building his own path toward career, friends, and his life. He knew the best way he could support his mother, and his father, was to not have them worried about him. He may have run out of the trust fund money, but he felt increasingly confident about his future, whatever that might be.

ASSESSMENT OF PROGRESS

Therapy is continuing on a weekly basis and Matt is able to note a number of changes that have occurred. His level of panic anxiety had all but vanished. This was particularly evident in his ability to talk about his father's cognitive decline and separate it from the maturational struggles of his mid twenties. A narrative understanding of current patterns enabled him to tolerate the ups and downs in his romantic relationship without behaving in self-defeating ways. And his overall sense of neediness toward those around him decreased and was replaced by a more positive, realistic appraisal of his strengths and weaknesses. While he still struggles with career-oriented occupational pursuits, he is at least being sensible with his expectations. Rather than focusing on having squandered his trust fund, he began to focus on what he hoped to accomplish in the future. This hope was genuine and more grounded in reality, compared with the intense fears of the future he came to therapy with. Even the guilt he had experienced when he spoke about the trust fund was more balanced and less self-critical. While he still regretted how he had spent some of it, he looked back on the past as a learning experience in the value of money and hard work.

Matt's crippling morning paralysis had been vanquished by psychotherapy and a three times a week gym membership, and a couple of new dogs represented an end to his wandering ways and a thought out decision to take on new responsibility. His overall mood had improved and lifted and seemed more resilient to rejection. His sense of humor and lightheartedness were more easily expressed and seemed to come from a newfound comfort in himself. Matt said he knew he would still encounter self-doubt and insecurity, but he also knew he was strong enough to manage these feelings himself.

While termination has not come up in treatment yet, we will need to be mindful of possible dependency on me. One day recently, Matt came in wearing that stiff-brimmed black hat again. I realized that while it had been a constant in therapy for many months, and I had not seen it for a while. I pointed out that he rarely wore it anymore. In college, when he first started to go prematurely bald, he was so ashamed that he rarely went out without a hat. He feared it made him look old. But he smiled and chuckled a little bit as he removed it and ran his hand over a smoothly shaven baldhead. "I don't really care that I'm bald anymore. Actually, I think it looks good." He smiled confidently as he ran his hand back over his head. Keeping the hat off, he gazed momentarily out the window. It was raining, but somehow, the lighting on Matt's face made him appear not just brighter, but truly alive.

CHAPTER 12

HORRIFIED AND GUILTY
A Case of Panic Anxiety

DHWANI SHAH

Adam, a 60-year-old man who left an unhappy marriage and is on the verge of moving in with his girlfriend, came to treatment for an exacerbation of panic attacks. This case is especially interesting because of the extensive direct quotes of the interaction between the patient and therapist. You can feel the patient's anxiety and distress and his increasing openness and relief over the course of the treatment.

A 3-month treatment was planned and the therapist pursues a focus on core conflicts about separation, loss, and fear that anger will lead to loss. This topic is taken up over and over, and the therapy proceeds as the therapist's gentle but firm approach brings these feelings and conflicts into the open and encourages their deeper exploration. Ultimately, interpretations bring the patient significant relief. This case provides a wonderful example of what is referred to in psychodynamic therapy as "working from the surface." This means starting with what the patient knows and feels most clearly (the surface) and gently working to extend the patient's awareness further and further as he or she gets more and more comfortable (the depth).

The patient asks for more guidance and advice, a frequent phenomenon in psychodynamic therapy, and the therapist interprets this in the context of the patient's transference reaction. There is an extended discussion of these feelings and detailed examples of how a therapist can inquire about transference and discuss it directly.

CHIEF COMPLAINT AND PRESENTATION

When I first met Adam, I was struck more by his fatigue than by his anxiety. He was a Polish laboratory technician in his early 60s with a full head of grey hair and dressed casually in jeans and a comfortable sweatshirt. He appeared emotionally exhausted and weakened by his current situation and spoke softly but curtly with only occasional eye contact. Despite his somewhat distancing demeanor, his gentle presence gave me the impression of a man who was sensitive and thoughtful. Adam wanted to start therapy because of disabling panic attacks that had been worsening over the past several months, particularly at work. He was especially concerned that his symptoms would impact his ability to work and provide for his family.

Adam's first disabling panic attack occurred 6 months before seeing me, when he was confronted by his manager for not keeping up with his expected workload. Shortly before then, he had been promoted to a new position at work in charge of specific lab orders, because several of his colleagues had unexpectedly left. Sally, his new manager, told Adam in a "matter of fact tone" that if he did not "shape up," she would have to reduce his hours and possibly demote him. Adam already felt overwhelmed by his demands at work and at home. Many of the coworkers that he used to rely on for help either had left the company or were on sick leave. He found himself lost in his new position and did not know whom he could turn to for help or support. The day of his first panic attack at work coincided with his girlfriend Joan and his son, Ian, moving to his new home. He still had not told his ex-wife Sarah about the move. "It would kill her," he suggested. Ian, 19 years old, was struggling. He had failed out of community college he was attending and was living at home, spending endless hours online. Adam suspected Ian was depressed or using drugs, and he got angry and defensive whenever Adam attempted to speak to him.

HISTORY

Adam had recently gone through a "hellish" marital separation that was still ongoing. He and his ex-wife Sarah had separated 1 year earlier, but Adam was still struggling with a profound sense of guilt and remorse for leaving his wife. He described Sarah as a "stern and emotionally removed person" who "holds a grudge." Sarah struggled with depression and had been hospitalized for a suicide attempt early in their marriage. Adam often worried about her and took on the burden of providing for the family and doing chores around the house to help her. His older son,

Tim, was 25 years old and in a successful career as an engineer. Ian, by contrast, struggled and often had screaming matches with Sarah, which led them both to agree that Ian should live with Adam. At that time Adam was in a relationship with a new woman, Joan, but was keeping this a secret from Sarah. He had recently moved into a new house and felt pressure to have Joan live with him, but was terrified of Ian's and Sarah's reactions to this.

Adam described classic panic symptoms during moments where he recalled tensions between himself and Sarah—rapid heart rate, intense sweating, and a fear that he was going to die or lose his mind. He had a feeling of unreality, as if "I am shrinking and everything around me is getting larger." He occasionally took alprazolam (prescribed by his internist) when he had these attacks, and felt it helped, but felt it also made him feel lightheaded and "out of sorts." A physical exam and lab work done by his internist demonstrated slightly high blood pressure and a mildly elevated pulse, but no other significant issues.

Although Adam could identify confrontations and the possibly of hurting others as triggers for his anxiety, he also described feeling frightened that an attack could occur at any time and would catch him off guard. Sometimes his anxiety came "out of the blue" when he was ruminating about his responsibilities at work or watching TV. During these moments, he had thoughts about confrontations with his boss or his son, his financial stressors and intrusive thoughts about death and dying, including thoughts that his car could swerve out of control and he could get into a horrific crash. He felt frightened about hurting people and did everything possible in order not to anger or upset others. He felt crushed when people he cared for were hurt or upset. He tearfully remembered his wife yelling "selfish bastard" at him, and feeling horrified and guilty over leaving her. Looking at me, he added, "But I needed a change, I couldn't survive living that way."

Despite Sarah being intelligent and loyal, Adam felt she was chronically emotionally unavailable to him. He related stories of her constant complaining, health issues, isolative behaviors, and angry outbursts. He felt she was self-centered and never cared about who he really was. In our first session together, Adam added that he felt Sarah was in many ways like his mother, chronically emotionally unavailable and self-involved, thinking about her needs before anyone else's.

In the first few weeks of therapy, Adam related more about his childhood to me. Adam often felt alone and unprotected growing up. It seemed to him danger was always lurking somewhere. He grew up in a working class family near Pittsburgh with his younger brother and his parents. His father worked in construction and was chronically unhappy about his job, often coming home sullen and distant. Adam described him as a kind and gentle man, and he remembered warm moments between the two of them fondly when Adam was 4 years old. But, as Adam grew up, he experienced his father as more of a distant and sullen figure, often quietly drinking beer alone listening to sports radio. This behavior often angered Adam's mother, whom he described as a "screamer . . . an intense woman."

Adam's mother was a formidable presence in the household, feared by Adam and his brother. She screamed at them for no clear reason, and Adam felt "there was always calm before the storm, the storm being my mother. Even when things were quiet, I was scared. I knew something would go wrong and all hell would break loose. I wonder if that's why my father became more distant, he couldn't stand it anymore."

Because he experienced his mother as emotionally threatening, Adam took on the responsibility of caring for his brother, who was fragile and often physically ill. At the age of 9, Adam's brother was diagnosed with diabetes and needed insulin injections daily. Adam remembered feeling constantly worried that his brother could die if he did not get his injections. School was also difficult for Adam. He remembered feeling unsafe away from home and felt other children at school judged him because of his ethnic background and limited means. At the age of 10, Adam moved to another school district in a lower income neighborhood after his father lost his job as a construction manager. Although his parents were disappointed in the new school system and its lack of resources, Adam thrived there because he was able to meet friends there and feel less alone.

Adam met Sarah in high school, and she was his first true love. Sarah became pregnant with their first son at the age of 20 and the two decided to marry. "I was young, but ready to settle down. All I wanted was to have a close family, a family where we all did things together, where things wouldn't get ruined all the time. I hoped for camping and hiking together, going on family trips, and building a family life together. That's what I wanted with Sarah. I think she wanted it too, and for a few years things were good, but then her depression began and she became distant. There was nothing I felt I could do, I felt trapped. I ended up doing everything for the family—working full time, paying all the bills, taking care of both of our children. . . . I feel like she didn't do anything. Although I wore a smile to everyone, I was dead inside. Thinking about this makes me feel lightheaded, almost like I am having an attack."

But, Adam also felt overwhelmed by his new life with Joan, as well as his new house and his new job responsibilities. Despite feeling Joan was a more nurturing, caring person than his wife, he could not help but miss Sarah. "I feel this guilt and sadness about it, but it's more like I don't feel like this new life is mine. My heart started racing and I felt funny the minute I started thinking about Joan moving into the new house. It's like this is not my life, and this does not feel right. But she is right for me in so many ways, we do things, meet people, and she's kind to me—this is the most caring a person has been toward me in my whole life. Why do I feel so anxious about it?"

CORE PSYCHODYNAMIC PROBLEM AND FORMULATION

Part I: Summarizing Statement

Adam was a 60-year-old divorced man with panic attacks associated with losses, life transitions, and fears of hurting others emotionally. He struggled as a child with fears about his mother's unpredictable anger and a sense of aloneness. He is struggling with transitioning to living with his new girlfriend and fears his former wife's angry reaction to this decision.

Part II: Description of Nondynamic Factors

Adam met the DSM-5 criteria for panic disorder. Although he did not know a great deal about his paternal or maternal grandparents, he reported his mother struggled with lifelong anxiety and depression, and his father he felt was depressed and used alcohol in an abusive manner. Adam was an anxious and shy young boy and often felt frightened of being left and unprotected, which may in part have been due to his anxious temperament.

His only prior therapy was couple therapy with his wife prior to the separation; he felt he could not be emotionally honest in that treatment. Although he used alprazolam on occasion with some benefit, he was skeptical of medications and wanted to come to terms with his anxiety in therapy. He had a medical history of high blood pressure and high cholesterol, which were actively being treated with a beta blocker and a statin.

Part III: Psychodynamic Explanation of Central Conflicts

I felt Adam's core psychodynamic issue was panic anxiety. His main conflicts centered on his early sense of abandonment and his anger and guilt associated with becoming his own person. Because of his vulnerability to anxiety, possibly due to a family history of mood disorders and an anxious temperament, he was especially sensitive to his early emotional distance from his mother and her unavailability, as well as her anger. I also saw Adam as highly conflicted about his angry feelings toward the people he cares about, and ambivalent about his wish to be an independent man.

It seemed that in early childhood Adam had developed the fear that fully experiencing his anger and separateness would cause him to lose whatever closeness he felt from his mother. He was able to express his dependency needs through helping his younger brother and his ex-wife, Sarah. He was a caretaker, identifying with those he was caring for, but his identification with those he cared for was costly because he felt secretly resentful and frustrated over not being cared for himself and not having his needs attended to. He also may have experienced his anger as too closely identified with his mother's rage, which terrified him. Adam's inhibited anger and resentment seemed to provoke more fears of abandonment and separation because of his fear that his anger would hurt the very people he depended on and cause a further rupture. A vicious cycle was created: Adam cares for his loved ones in the way that he secretly wants to be cared for, but then feels unappreciated and mistreated when he does not get this caring back in return. His resentment and anger about this mistreatment then frightens him and causes him to feel guilty and alone, which increases his anxiety and leads to more caretaking, which then leads to more resentment. This emotional pattern also caused Adam to see himself as vulnerable and fragile and this increased his fears about expressing his autonomy and his assertiveness.

This cycle of caretaking and resentment also occurred in his marriage to Sarah. The need to take care of her to avoid conflict resulted in the split. In his new relationship with Joan, he found a woman whom he felt could love in the way he always wanted. But, being with her meant losing his old familiar love relationships and hurting them, about which he felt very guilty. Not telling Sarah about the move allowed him a safe space to express his aggression toward her without confronting her or feeling guilt in a split off fashion. That is, he knew that not telling her in advance would make her more angry.

I felt it was important that his first panic attack occurred when he was about to move in to his new house. Not only were his assertiveness and anger expressed clearly in this act by abandoning his ex-wife Sarah, but it was a moment of autonomy. Adam cannot bear to feel sadness, anger, or guilt, so when they arise, he experiences panic. His panic symptoms expressed his unbearable fear of loss and defensively dealt with the anger to maintain a position of weakness and fragility which felt less threatening.

Adam had a number of strengths as well. He was obviously a compassionate individual who loved and cared for others, and he had a number of supportive friends. Despite his conflicts with his family, he also maintained a good relationship with his younger brother and his eldest son. He also frequently saw and felt close to his aging father, with whom he felt quite close despite his struggling with dementia. When he was not burdened by sadness and anxiety, he described himself as energetic, fun loving, and spontaneous. He was intelligent and hardworking and performed well at his job when he was not suffering from anxiety.

Part IV: Predicting Responses to the Therapeutic Situation

Adam has many positive prognostic features for psychotherapy. He is quite symptomatic but high-functioning, honest, and open. I felt he would likely want to avoid the painful feelings of loss and anger, and fear over loss of control of his anger that is apparent in his relationships. Behavioral and psychological avoidance of these difficult emotions will probably be an important theme in the therapy and will have to be addressed in order for him to make progress. It is also possible that the dynamics of his relationship with Sarah could arise in his relationship with me. He may avoid his angry feelings and his assertiveness in the room with me in fear of potentially damaging our relationship, and experience that anger instead as anxiety. So, he will avoid being direct with me, feel angry at me for not helping him, yet be reluctant to explore those feelings. He may also become very attached and fear the loss of the treatment when it ultimately ends.

COURSE OF TREATMENT

Adam's psychotherapy first focused on the precipitants to panic attacks, and this led to deeper discussions of his feelings of loss, dependency, anger, and fear of expressing anger and avoidance of controversy. We worked on his anxiety around assertiveness in relation to the authority figures in his life, and his attitude in the therapy sessions, and then moved on to discuss his conflicted feelings about his mother. Adam's feelings about our relationship were a focus, especially later in the treatment, and his feelings of anger and guilt were played out in his feelings about me. His panic symptoms subsided as he became more aware of these issues and how they were triggered in his everyday life.

Initially, based on Adam's slowed body language and nervous tone of voice, I could sense Adam's sadness and worry about the state of his current life. Although he did not appear clinically depressed, he clearly was sad and his mood was low. He said he felt depleted and guilty about his work situation and where his life was going. The symptoms that troubled him most, however, were his panic attacks and his frequent worry about having more symptoms. His panic attacks felt physically uncomfortable to him and had an unsettling visceral quality to them—the lightheadedness, heart palpitations, sweating, and feeling of unreality made him extremely uncomfortable and were difficult to bear. The unpredictability of the episodes troubled him and left him feeling helpless and anxious about when they would happen. Although he felt many of the attacks occurred out of the blue, he was usually able to point out specific thoughts and feelings he was having prior to the episodes.

Many of Adam's triggers seemed to involve his guilt about being assertive with those in authority who upset or frustrated him. He appeared to have difficulty in setting limits with others and putting into words his own need to be cared for and comforted. Adam seemed to put other people's needs before his while feeling resentful about this.

We agreed after our first several meetings that Adam would benefit from twice weekly psychotherapy. Although he was burdened with panic symptoms and sadness, he was thoughtful and able to connect his words with his experiences and emotions. He was able to identify patterns from his past and connect them with his present circumstances in an emotionally meaningful manner.

Adam gave verbal agreement to start therapy with me but his body language indicated more doubt. Although he described himself as outgoing and extroverted he appeared reticent and somewhat removed, with little eye contact, often gazing at my bookshelf or the clock. When speaking about his past and his anger toward Sarah, he often nervously laughed and rubbed the back of his head. In our first several sessions together, I found myself having a difficult time emotionally understanding what Adam was saying. He spoke quickly, often giving me minute details about the way in which the technical equipment in the office worked and how the office was set up to handle medical issues. He seemed more comfortable talking with me about what he knew and was competent at than about his emotional life.

Adam was under a tremendous amount of emotional strain. He had left his wife and his old position at work, his son was struggling to find a path for himself and was angry and depressed, and he was living miles away from his old neighborhood. As he related this to me, I felt the gravity of the loss of his comfortable way of life and how difficult that loss was for him to bear. Despite his past frequent daydreaming about a new life, Adam was terribly frightened about his new reality and its emotional significance. He was also carrying a tremendous amount of guilt over breaking up his marriage and its effects on his wife and his son.

I began to feel that Adam's emotionally distanced way of relating to me in our sessions was a compromise between his wish to honestly relate what he was experiencing and his need to ward off the sadness, anger, and guilt he was experiencing about this transition. I felt his panic symptoms were directly related to this compromise. Whenever these difficult feelings threatened to break the surface, especially if they involved him being separate from his comfortable old surroundings and being autonomous, his panic symptoms emerged.

When he walked near his department in the hospital where he used to work, Adam related feeling "this weird sensation like I am about to have a panic attack, I feel myself shrinking and everything around me getting bigger and moving. My heart starts to race and I feel like I'm going to lose control, like I am going to collapse or something." I asked him if any of these symptoms were occurring as he was relating this to me. He replied that he often felt these symptoms when he talked about them, but "I try really hard not to feel them. It feels really uncomfortable, I can't stand feeling this way."

I told him that I could tell how terrible and out of control he felt with these sensations and added that although the symptoms were uncomfortable, the fact that he was feeling them in the moment gave us the opportunity to understand what they meant to him. "None of this feels right," he replied. "My new job, my new house, living with Joan—I feel I should feel happy but I don't. This is hard to talk about. I'm feeling dizzy just thinking about it."

I suggested to Adam that perhaps the somatic symptoms he was experiencing were about this sudden change and what it meant to him. "Damn it! I didn't want my life to go this way. I miss the family we had, I miss Sarah," he said tearfully. "I never wanted this to happen. I wanted to have a new life, a new beginning, but not like this. I think I wanted it with Sarah. I love Joan, I feel really guilty for saying this, she is so good to me, but I feel this is all too different. And my son isn't doing anything. He sits all day on the computer playing video games, not applying to schools or trying to get a job. It's like he doesn't care, and I've been a failure as a parent. I should have kept things the way they were." I replied that it seemed that these uncomfortable sensations and anxiety occurred when he was feeling the consequences of his new life and being more independent. I added that it seemed that whenever he allowed himself to feel this new independence he felt guilty, which seemed to fuel his anxiety as well. Tearfully he agreed and said that he felt guilty about everything, and that this guilt has been there his whole life. "But I have reason to feel it," he added. "Look at what I've done to my son. But I just couldn't live with her anymore, it was horrible. The yelling, the arguing, there was no fun, we never did anything fun together. With Joan I feel I have a new life."

"Notice the shift," I said, "from talking about feeling unbearably guilty and feeling it was all your fault to speaking of your need to leave, for yourself and your son. It feels like you are really uncomfortable with feeling guilty and asserting what it is you need and desire. You are constantly trying to fight off feeling guilty and perhaps wanting others, like me, to make you feel less guilty."

"I've never done anything like this before," he replied. "This is brand new. And it all doesn't feel right. I've been with Sarah this whole time, managing everything, her moods and her illness, hating it. But I guess it was comfortable on some strange level, because I never felt anxiety like this until now."

Adam arrived at his next session reporting he was feeling somewhat better. Although he had not had a full-blown panic attack, he still felt uncomfortable being at work with his new boss, Sally. She continued to place demands on him that he felt were unrealistic. It made him feel she was critical of him and his abilities. Discussing it further, he added that she had told him not to be so hard on himself, and to "take it one day at a time." Noticing this change in his description of Sally, I asked him if he felt some of what he was experiencing as disapproval and criticism from Sally may be the pressure and guilt he feels for not pleasing her or doing what he was asked. He paused and said, "I'm not sure, but maybe. The feeling does in some ways remind me of what it was like with my ex-wife, Sarah. I felt like she was constantly telling me I wasn't doing enough for her, but I really was in reality. It's like I feel guilty all the time. I think I feel guilty for my very existence—whenever I want something for myself that could be something that would upset someone else. Being with Joan, living this new life, this is for me. But it doesn't feel right."

Adam went on to describe the difficult financial situation he was in. After Sarah stopped working because of depression, Adam began to take on all of the finances for his family, and the bills began to pile up. Slowly, without telling Sarah, certain bills were not paid because there was no money. Eventually, paying for the mortgage was delayed and the house was threatened with foreclosure. "I never mentioned any of this to Sarah. When she found out, she was so upset with me. I've never seen her so out of control. I think I didn't tell her because I can't stand hurting her, she was so upset and depressed already. I didn't want to make things worse."

When I asked what it was about confrontation that was so difficult for him, he described feeling totally anxious and undone. "I can't stand it. It is like the panic sensations but in some ways worse. I just want to run and hide." When I pressed him on what felt dangerous, he said that it almost felt like he was going to die, or something horrible was going to happen.

"I notice that you often speak of others being angry or upset with you and your being frightened by this, but you don't often speak of your own angry feelings," I replied. He paused and went on to talk about how difficult it is for him to feel his anger. "I always feel someone is going to get hurt or something like that. Getting angry means hurting someone, and that doesn't feel right to me."

I replied, "I wonder if this relates to the panic symptoms. It seems like you are really uncomfortable with angry feelings or being assertive. Someone is going to get hurt and this is really scary for you. The panic symptoms seem to take you away from these angry feelings."

He went on to talk about work and his boss. "I know she probably means well, but I can't stand her, and it's true—I feel anxious just thinking about her and the things she says. I just want to avoid her, but I admit I've had lots of angry thoughts about her. She is always trying to boss me around and she doesn't even really understand the nuances of what I do, she just watches and comments."

As he related this to me, I remembered his resentment toward his mother for being unavailable to him and for being a "screamer." I asked him if he felt his angry feelings were frightening for him growing up. He shook his head and replied, "I can't get over how irresponsible my mother was toward me. She was so wound up, so unhappy all the time. I felt she was always checked out and left me to take care of everything, including my brother. And I can't talk to her about it now. She's one of those people who can never apologize or own anything. She would just deny it. I remember getting really anxious about picking up my son on time for school, as if I am 5 minutes late, something horrible was going to happen. I think I'm anxious about it because that is what happened to me all the time. I remember just sitting there waiting for her to come get me, not knowing when she would show up. I would be the last kid sitting there. And then there were days at a time when I would be left at the babysitter's house, why I still don't know. I remember having to pick up cigarettes and food for my babysitter, walking by myself unprotected. I must have been 10 years old."

When I asked what that was like, he said with a laugh, "I was alone. Always fending for myself." Reflecting on his ability to ward off feelings by using humor, I said: "I notice you are laughing, but what you are describing sounds like it was incredibly painful to you."

He replied, "I think it makes me really mad and upset, but I feel like that's difficult for me to feel, so I just laugh it off. But you are right, it really doesn't sound that funny." He then remembered an incident that "still bothers me at my core to this day." He and his brother were playing with a baseball inside his house and he accidentally threw the ball at an old clock on a mantle in the living room. The clock shattered, waking up his mother who was taking a nap upstairs. She raced down the stairs and screamed at both Adam and his brother to "get out." Frightened, they ran outside through the back door and his mother then locked the doors of the house and refused to let them come back inside. "I can't remember how long it was, but it felt like hours. My little brother, crying, wailing really, and I had to calm him down. I was so scared he was going to get sick or die of shock. After a while I realized I had to do something. I was able to climb through a window and I saw my mom there, just frozen, staring off into space. I took my brother upstairs and we just tried to forget it happened." We discussed how he was able to be assertive and take care of himself when it mattered most. Despite his fears of hurting others, he was capable of asserting his needs and protecting himself.

As Adam became more aware of the dynamics of his panic symptoms and deepened his understanding of his guilt about leaving his wife, the focus of the work shifted toward the transference. Even though we were meeting twice per week and his panic attacks were lessening, Adam began to seem more emotionally distant. At the end of a session, after talking about how overwhelmed he was by his son's passivity and inability to work toward a goal, he remarked that he would not be able to come in for our next session and needed to change the time. After agreeing to another time, he added, "Are you going to really help me with this? I mean, well, give me some tips or some guidance in how I should deal with this?"

The question surprised me and I realized that despite Adam's openness about many topics, he never spoke about how he felt the therapy was going or about any feelings toward me as his therapist. I replied, "That's a really important question, and one that I feel may have been difficult for you to ask. Let's talk about it more next time if it feels important to you." Although I did not say this, I felt his asking at the end of the session was a way of avoiding any conflict that this question generated. He laughed and said reassuringly he felt "really good" about coming in but felt he wanted more "skills" to manage the panic attacks.

Adam ended up missing his next two sessions with me. He called, apologetic, stating that his work was just too busy and he could not make time to come in. I speculated that some disappointment about the therapy and me were coming up that made him feel uncomfortable. Avoiding the sessions in a friendly manner seemed to be a way of avoiding any confrontation with me. Ten days later when he arrived at his appointment 15 minutes late, he apologized again. When I asked about how he felt about missing the sessions, he quickly brushed passed the question and said he was "really busy but overall doing well."

When I pressed him a bit further, however, he added, "I sometimes don't know if I am doing things right in here. You don't give me a direction to go in, and I feel like maybe I'm just doing this wrong or something."

I asked him about the missed sessions and if they had to do with these feelings, and he reluctantly said, "See, there it is again, doc. I think I feel judged by you, like I'm not doing it right. I feel like that right now, like you are giving me trouble for not coming in . . . although I know that's not what you are really doing, I feel that way." I appreciated Adam's honesty about this and acknowledged that to him. Examining my own feelings privately, I did notice some worry and annoyance about the missed sessions.

Still, it appeared he was warding off an attack and playing it safe. He constantly felt judged and frightened about his feelings, and how others would receive them. Reflecting on how Adam often projected his feelings of guilt on to others, I said, "It seems that is a theme that is reoccurring between us. You often feel guilty about how you are feeling and need approval from others. Perhaps this sense of being judged by me is a way of expressing your own guilt and criticism of yourself and your inner life."

"I feel like I work really hard to get people to like me, and I end up getting tied in knots worrying about it to the point where I forget what I am feeling," he replied. "It's like I need to make sure others are OK before I am OK." Adam commented that he felt he needed to do this with his younger brother constantly. "Did this occur with anyone else in your life growing up?" I asked. "Well, I'm not sure, but for some reason this memory is coming up. I remember my father, coming home one day, angry and sullen as he often was. He went upstairs and I could hear my mom yelling at him. It felt horrible, as if there was a knot in my stomach. I don't know or remember where my brother Tommy was. I went upstairs and stood by the door, listening to my father sobbing, wailing. He wasn't okay, and I couldn't do anything to help him."

A memory of angrily rebuking his father for not coming to his middle school softball game emerged. After this confrontation, he was frightened by his father's reaction. Surprisingly, his father, instead of punishing him, sat helplessly and just shook his head silently. Adam remembered feeling terribly frightened and overwhelmed with guilt. "I think I panic when I think about how much my father has disappointed me in not helping me be stronger."

"Perhaps it is because of a sense of him being so fragile. It seems if you have any negative or angry thoughts toward him, you feel anxious and guilt-ridden. Perhaps this also helps us understand why it is difficult for you to allow yourself to be critical of me—in those moments you see me as fragile as well, like you felt your father was.

Adam went on to say again that he had hoped for more direction and guidance in therapy. "I want to feel like I am making the right decision, and that I have a way of controlling my anxiety." I told Adam that his concerns about wanting a direction and more instruction on treating his panic symptoms were understandable, considering the distress he was experiencing. However, it seemed that having me "tell him what to do" was also a way of avoiding painful feelings. It seemed in order for him to feel safe, Adam felt he had to do what he imagined others wanted him to do. I suggested he needed to become more comfortable in being his own person.

Adam began the next session by talking about his son and how miserable he was at home. He felt anxious when his son confronted him about the move and made demands about it. "I feel I need to make him happy, do what is best for him, and if I don't he gets really mad and sullen. He starts accusing me of not being a good dad, messing up the family, that it's my fault he can't get his act together, and I start to feel overwhelmed and uncomfortable. I get dizzy and my head spins. It's like the anxiety comes back in a flash." When I inquired more about the details of what he was thinking and feeling in these moments, Adam said he felt attacked in those moments and felt like he was a terrible father. "He's right after all. It was my fault. I'm the one who left Sarah . . . and he needed me. I ruined the family. I think I get mad back at him, but then I think to myself, who am I to get mad? I just want him to be happy."

It seemed to be difficult for Adam to set limits and responsibilities with his son in a compassionate way. Whenever his son demanded something from him, he felt as though he needed to provide it, yet felt resentful in the process of doing so. This process seemed to fuel his guilt and made him feel more anxious, increasing his need to give his son what he wanted. Underneath his anger, however, it seemed Adam felt he needed to be everything for his son. Setting limits and being firm with him felt frightening to him. Adam allowed his son to live in their home with no expectations or limitations, and his son was struggling to be responsible for himself and others. By not allowing himself to experience his disappointment and sadness over his son's behavior, he realized that he actually was avoiding his son, and this was making the situation worse.

As time passed in treatment, the theme of caring for others emerged as central. Care giving seemed to help keep Adam feeling safe in relationships, but it also became clear that it was a way of avoiding painful feelings of being alone without a home base. Adam remembered with great feeling waiting by the door of his house, desperately waiting for his father to come home. "It was a gut wrenching experience, I felt out of control, dizzy. I can feel it now even. That horrible feeling of being left alone, with no one to protect or help you—it's like you can't even breathe." The panic symptoms seemed to be tied into a feeling of being abandoned without a "home base" and an available caregiver with whom he felt secure.

It felt important that these symptoms reoccurred after Adam began to make a transition to a new life with Joan. What was familiar to him was lost, and his new life felt without an anchor. "I failed everyone, my wife, my son, our family," Adam stated tearfully.

"It seems you feel you have spent your life living through what others want for you in order to feel safe. Living for yourself and making choices that are in your best interest threatens that security and leaves you vulnerable and with the panic symptoms," I said. Adam felt much better after this session and his anxiety throughout the week decreased, although it was difficult for him to identify why.

In subsequent sessions Adam talked more about his mixed feelings about his new life. "It's not perfect, Joan isn't what I pictured in many ways as the ideal wife, but she is good to me and my life is better with her. We do things together and I am able to feel close to her in some ways that I never could with Sarah. I don't have to feel like I need to take care of her. But I miss my old life, my family, and Sarah." Slowly his panic symptoms decreased with some sadness and a sense of loss. It seemed that the more Adam was able to speak about his ambivalence about his new life with Joan and talk openly about longing for the closeness and security he was not able to have as a young boy, the less his panic symptoms haunted him. He was more insightful about himself and more emotionally engaged in our sessions together, although he still experienced anxiety about his son not succeeding and guilt over his role as a father.

TERMINATION

When Adam and I first met, we both decided that his therapy would be time limited. He started therapy to stop his panic symptoms and was not interested in long-term work. He had a new house, a busy full-time job, and a son who needed his attention. He wanted to live his life without constantly worrying about having another panic attack out of the blue, and to be relieved of the symptoms of anxiety that were burdening him. We both decided to meet twice a week for 3 months, and agreed it would be longer if he felt his symptoms had not improved, or if he wanted to work on the major transitions that were going on in his life.

As we approached the 3-month mark, Adam felt he was ready to end therapy. His symptoms of panic had improved, although at times his anxiety returned, especially when he had confrontations with his boss at work or when his son neglected his responsibilities at home or fought with Joan. Importantly, he felt more comfortable with being assertive with others, and was beginning to feel more autonomous and comfortable with living a life that he felt suited him. He still felt guilty over many of the decisions he had made over the past several years, but his guilt caused him less distress and anxiety than it had before. When he spoke again about his wish to end therapy, I suggested we schedule an end date and have several sessions for Adam to work on his feelings about ending treatment. In these sessions, Adam seemed eager to marry Joan and did not seem to have any strong feelings about ending the therapy.

His anxiety was improved and he was looking forward to having more time in his busy schedule once he no longer had therapy appointments to keep. Adam's anxiety increased during the week prior to our end date. It was a difficult week for him. Sarah, his ex-wife, was demanding he address several complicated financial matters, and his son recently had a job opportunity that he squandered by not coming in on time for the second interview. Adam felt overwhelmed and felt frightened about the treatment ending. "I think maybe I was taking it for granted, or just eager to stop because things were going well. But now I can feel some fear about not having a place to talk about what is going on. I feel really nervous talking about it."

We were able to identify these anxiety symptoms as a way of expressing his feelings about ending. Like previous transitions and moves toward independence, the end of therapy marked another loss of safety that was frightening to him. Putting these fears into words, and understanding that the end of therapy was an important transition, helped Adam make sense of his experience.

Reflecting privately on my own feelings, I also felt sadness at the ending of our work together. I admired Adam for his strength and determination at creating a new life for himself and his son, and hoped that his symptoms would not get in the way of his continuing to build confidence in himself and determine what was best for him and his family.

ASSESSMENT OF PROGRESS

Understanding that his panic symptoms related to his difficulties with asserting himself and being independent helped Adam feel less out of control and helpless when the now-attenuated symptoms occurred. An essential aspect of his improvement was learning not to "fear fear." Adam had exhausted a great deal of time and energy trying to avoid feeling his panic symptoms by caring and submitting to others. This behavior led to temporary decreases in anxiety, but ultimately to him resenting others and feeling trapped by them, which then led to more anxiety and worry about losing them, and feeling alone and unprotected. Describing his symptoms of panic, allowing them to be felt and put into words in the room with me, and understanding why they occurred led to him feeling less frightened of his symptoms. He was able to become more comfortable with the sensations and feelings that before felt frightening and out of control. He was able to more realistically assess others' feelings and was less prone to attribute anger and disappointment in them. He modified his characteristic coping style and was able to assert himself more and be less of a reflexive caretaker.

Due to time limitations, and my focus on his panic symptoms, we left many other of Adam's internal experiences unexamined. I struggled to keep the focus on the meaning of his panic symptoms because those were the symptoms that impaired him. We only touched on Adam's conflicted feelings about his relationship with his father, who was extremely important to him. Adam's father was kind and loyal, but ultimately disappointing because of his inaccessibility and his inability to be assertive and set limits with others in a strong and controlled manner. We also did not fully explore Adam's possible wish for (and fear of) a strong paternal figure. There were probably unexamined guilty competitive feelings with other men and his mother, which may have had origins in Adam feeling less connected to his father despite his shortcomings. His early childhood experience of different socioeconomic and ethnic background from peers had a significant impact on his ability feel safe, but we didn't explore this, either.

While Adam and I were able to talk about several emotional themes that occurred in the transference, including his feeling of being judged by me and needing to feel I should take the lead in deciding what we spoke about, I think these themes could have been worked through in more detail. For example, we really only started to explore his wish for me to take control as a way of avoiding conflicts over him being independent and his ability to be assertive. I feel Adam would have had the opportunity to work on this in greater depth in a longer-term psychotherapy and this would have allowed him a space to talk more about feeling judged or needing control as ways of protecting himself against dangers of being intimate or close with others as well. Overall, I hoped the treatment had been helpful and hoped that this new life transition would offer Adam the opportunity to be more confident and emotionally secure.

CHAPTER 13

OUR THERAPEUTIC JOURNEY

A Case of Trauma

KARLA CAMPANELLA

This remarkable treatment of Helen, a young woman with hearing impairment, a traumatic past, and nonepileptic seizures, shows both the accomplishments and the disappointments of a psychotherapy pursued with great perseverance by both the patient and the therapist. The case history reveals how difficult it is to encourage a patient with a "medical" problem to receive psychiatric and psychological treatment, and the complexity of doing psychotherapy with a patient with hearing impairment. It is also a cautionary tale about employing prolonged exposure therapy with a hearing-impaired patient who did not have a safe living arrangement. Furthermore, it describes some of the issues involved in changing the approach from a cognitive-behavioral therapy such as prolonged exposure to psychodynamic therapy.

The therapist describes the unfolding of the treatment with this brave but vulnerable patient with great candor and self-reflectiveness. When the partially deaf patient loses all of her hearing, the therapist realizes the power of an enactment she has participated in, and becomes increasingly aware of the impact of the transference and countertransference on the treatment. This awareness provides an opportunity to connect with the patient on a deeper level. But, new life experiences bring about a regression in the patient's symptomatology and challenge the therapist in her assessment of the impact of the treatment. The openness and humility of the therapist ultimately helps her process the experience and come to a sense of resolution about her work with the patient.

I had a patient tell me once, "If I'm thinking it, it must be normal because I'm not crazy." Therein lies the first hurdle in practicing psychodynamic psychotherapy—getting the patient into treatment. Many people struggle with one of the six core psychodynamic problems. Unfortunately, however, seeking treatment at a psychiatrist's office is often viewed as crossing an invisible line from "normal" into "crazy." Psychodynamic psychotherapy exists on the plain in between. It clarifies that, in the complex dance that is the human condition, there are six basic issues that can trip us up. In psychotherapy, there are problem-focused interventions for each issue that can get us back on track. The thread that holds the work together, securing it against the pressures of stigma, is the therapeutic alliance. And when the opportunity presents, the therapeutic alliance is the thread that can guide a patient into treatment.

Those who seek treatment on their own find that psychodynamic psychotherapy clarifies their issues and provides problem-focused interventions to get them back on track. For others, the stigma of entering into psychiatric treatment stops them from scheduling the initial appointment. Sometimes, an opportunity presents to do a psychiatric evaluation in a medical setting. If a therapeutic connection occurs, the person may feel willing to risk stigma to enter into treatment in the mental health environment.

CHIEF COMPLAINT AND PRESENTATION

Such a therapeutic connection occurred when I was doing a rotation in an epilepsy clinic. I was charged with doing an initial intake for Helen. She presented to the clinic for an evaluation of seizures that had begun 8 years ago. The seizures had worsened such that she was unable to work or drive. She had been recently discharged after a second hospitalization and neurologic workup without a diagnosis. "They mostly happen when I am around strange men," she told me. She also offered that she had had increasing depression and anxiety. When I asked about trauma she reported that she had experienced sexual abuse as both a child and an adult, and physical abuse from an ex-husband. I diverted from the neurological evaluation briefly to inquire about posttraumatic stress disorders (PTSD) symptoms. Indeed she was experiencing intrusive thoughts and nightmares, and she avoided situations associated with traumatic experiences.

After completing the neurologic evaluation, I explained to Helen that the neurologist would now come and determine the plan for addressing the seizures. However, since I was a psychiatrist-in-training, I could offer her separate treatment for her depression, anxiety, and trauma-associated symptoms. Although a psychiatric consultant had started her on medications during her last hospital stay, she had never been in treatment. She considered. I later realized how great the barriers were for her to come to see me. It meant crossing from a medical clinic to a psychiatric clinic, crossing state lines by train to get to the office each visit, and crossing the carefully erected perimeter her family had maintained to protect their secrets. I gave her my contact information, and then the neurologist came and concluded the visit. Weeks later, Helen showed up in my office and she told me her story.

HISTORY

Helen was born in a small town. Her father was well known as someone successful in his line of work. Her mother was known for her involvement in community activities. She had a brother several years older than her. She, however, was born partially deaf. Her parents were unable to accept the fact that she was different. Her mother learned some sign language, but her father refused. Her mother sent her to the local school that had no accommodations for hearing-impaired students. When Helen told her mother about difficulties at school her mother told her she just had to work harder to make up for her disability. Helen grew up believing that she must fit into the hearing world or she would be abandoned by her family.

Around the age of 4, a male speech therapist came to the house. He regularly molested her. Around that time also, her father began to molest her. From that point on, she refused to wear dresses. The physical and sexual abuse from her father continued—fueled by his heavy drug habit. Helen's mother regularly left the house to spend time with friends. Helen's brother would watch him abuse her but offer no help.

Helen would frequently revisit one memory from her childhood. She described how one evening her father was "high out of his mind" so she knew he would come after her. Her mother announced that she was leaving to visit friends at a park. Helen begged her mother to take her along to the park. Her mother refused and left. Helen was desperate to get out of the house. She began screaming and banging on the door. At one point her hand went through the glass, cutting her arm very badly. She stared at the blood and felt an overwhelming sense of relief because she wanted desperately to die and felt that it was now going to happen. At this point, her brother panicked and ran to the park and brought back her mother. Her parents argued loudly about taking her to the emergency room for stitches. In the end, her father refused to allow her mother to take her to the hospital. She had to visit the school nurse several times a day to change the dressing but the nurse overlooked the unusual nature of her injuries. Each time Helen told the story, she spoke about how angry she was at her brother for getting her mother and preventing her from being allowed to die. Helen grew up feeling that people were untrustworthy or dangerous and that she was powerless in the face of a school and family committed to keeping secrets.

To cope with these stresses, Helen began to drink heavily at a young age. She often stayed out in the woods until late to avoid being home with her father. She often drank at parties with other groups of teenagers. However, Helen clarified, she arrived at the parties already drunk and was not there to socialize but to escape from what was waiting at home. When it was time for Helen to choose a college, she went to one that did not make accommodations for her hearing impairment. Nevertheless, she managed to graduate from college while still drinking heavily. After Helen graduated and got a job, she stopped using alcohol as a coping strategy.

Around the time that Helen stopped drinking, she began to have "shaking spells" at work. She started seeing multiple neurologists and had two hospital admissions over several years to evaluate these episodes. Under pressure from her mother, she married a man from church. He was physically abusive, and after 2 years she escaped under cover of darkness and returned home. Her mother was angry with her for leaving him, saying that marriage should be a lifetime commitment. Helen did not tell her that he had been physically abusive.

At the time that Helen entered therapy, she was living with a female friend from high school. She felt stressed in that living situation because her friend drank heavily and had many male friends who would come to the apartment intoxicated. Helen felt unsafe there, especially because her father abused her while he was intoxicated. Shortly after starting therapy, Helen moved out while her roommate was out of town. She eventually moved back into her old room at her parent's house.

When Helen presented to our office she was seeking help for two troubling symptoms: anger and numbness. She had no understanding that these were characteristic responses to trauma. Instead these symptoms made her feel ashamed and empty. She reported that others often commented to her that she was an "angry child" when she was growing up. She felt ashamed of this. She said she remembers becoming angry and acting out in school when she knew her father was due to return from a business trip. She reported intense anger toward her brother, who had watched the abuse and turned away. She currently felt anger toward her brother's children because they were starting to get into legal trouble and bring shame to the family. She was angry at her mother because although as a child she begged her to leave her father, her mother refused. When Helen left her own abusive marriage, her mother blamed Helen for "not trying hard enough" to stay in the marriage. Helen was angry that both of her parents had managed to remain respectable and successful at work and in the community despite what had happened in their home. At times this anger would boil over into outbursts and Helen did not like the way these outbursts made her feel out of control.

Helen's most troubling symptom, however, was a pervasive numbness. She reported that she remembered very little of her childhood and this bothered her. She was able to see others around her experiencing a range of emotions but she could not seem to feel emotions herself. At times, especially when she was around strange men, people who were yelling, or people using substances, she would feel fear. But often she could not identify the emotion as fear and would say she felt "restless." She was unable to feel pleasant emotions, such as joy or contentment. She knew she wanted to stop feeling numb but she did not know how to do it.

Helen frequently expressed anger that her family refused to accept her hearing impairment. Her mother had learned some American Sign Language (ASL) but preferred not to use it. Her father refused to learn ASL. Because her family attempted to deny her deafness, she developed a way of relating to the world as if she had full hearing. Rather than draw attention to her hearing impairment, she would pretend that she understood what was going on around her even if she did not. This meant she refused all assistive devices despite the consequences of increased dependence on her mother. She went to a college where she was the only hearing-impaired person, despite reporting frustration at being made to attend a secondary school where she was the only deaf child. These choices by her parents also had implications for how Helen had been accepted by the deaf community. Because Helen is not fluent in ASL and mainly communicates verbally, she labeled herself as "oral deaf." Historically, there has been a long and contentious debate in the deaf community between advocates of oralism and those who advocate manual communication (Steinberg, 1991). Helen reported to me that she felt stigmatized by the deaf community because she felt that most of the deaf people she met were manual communicators and rejected her for communicating verbally. Helen described herself as always on the periphery—not fully part of the hearing world due to her deafness, and not fully part of the hearing-impaired world because she was verbal.

Helen struggled with defining her identity and personal boundaries. She had never lived alone. At the times when she moved out of her parent's home, she would live with others who caused her to feel unsafe. At the time we began therapy, she was in the process of leaving a roommate who was a substance abuser in order to move back in with her parents. Helen reported that she did not feel unsafe moving back to the same home with her father because he had stopped abusing her and using substances. Because Helen did not identify herself as deaf, she did not utilize the telephone equipment and occupational training available to her. This resulted in difficulty in using the phone and limited her ability to find work. She relied on others, especially her mother, to communicate if she could not use text messaging. She chose to identify exclusively with the hearing world as a means of staying connected with her family. This resulted in difficulty understanding what was happening around her. She also depended on her mother to make phone calls. This allowed her mother to know all the details of Helen's life so that she had no privacy. Helen refused any assistive devices because, while they would allow her to live independently, they would define her as deaf.

CORE PSYCHODYNAMIC PROBLEM AND FORMULATION

As we settled in to start the work of therapy, I already knew enough about Helen's experiences to start with a working formulation.

Part I: Summarizing Statement

Helen was a middle-aged woman with difficulty identifying and expressing her feelings (alexithymia), emotional numbing, frequent episodes of disassociation which included seizure-like shaking of her head and limbs, a history of alcohol dependence, and chronic low-grade depression. These symptoms interfered with her ability to work and live independently. Helen experienced sexual and physical abuse when she was young and had a tendency to become involved in situations that caused further trauma, such as marrying a physically abusive man. Helen was afraid to be around people involved with substance abuse because her father abused her when he was under the influence of substances. However, one of her most recent housing situations involved others living in the household who abused substances.

Helen reported a great longing for independence and a satisfying job. Although she had worked in caring for special needs children in the past, she had mixed feelings about caring for children. She found that she had trouble relating to them and would lose her patience easily.

Part II: Description of Nondynamic Factors

Helen's ability to hear was 70% below normal, but she was able to supplement her deficit by lip reading. She meets diagnostic criteria for PTSD. Because the trauma occurred at a young developmental age and persisted throughout childhood, Helen is predisposed to mood disorders. The fact that she drank heavily throughout her teen years also interfered with normal adolescent psychosocial development. Her mother's depression predisposes her genetically and developmentally through neglect to a mood disorder. The fact that her father was a heavy substance user suggests that Helen may have a genetic susceptibility to misuse alcohol. Because her father abused her throughout childhood when he was under the influence of substances, Helen has ongoing PTSD symptoms of arousal and reexperiencing when she is exposed to substance abuse in others.

Part III: Psychodynamic Explanation of Central Conflicts

The core psychodynamic problem Helen faces is trauma. Because she had experienced early and persistent threats to her safety, she was hypervigilant and easily triggered by environmental cues.

The traditional psychodynamic understanding of nonepileptic seizures is that they are an outward manifestation of inner psychic conflict. The physical symptoms act to communicate distress and escape the mental conflict. These symptoms may also be unconsciously chosen because they elicit attention and sympathy when expressing the mental conflict directly would likely cause a negative reaction in those around them (Nowak & Fink, For Helen, the nonepileptic seizures were a way of communicating the inner distress that she had trouble expressing. These shaking episodes also caused her family and friends to be attentive to her. The family did not allow Helen to discuss or seek support related to her father's abuse. She often expressed frustration at having to carry on with all the small-town activities as if she came from a model family. But epilepsy was a topic that was easy to discuss both in public and in private.

Part IV: Predicting Responses to the Therapeutic Situation

I anticipated that the nonepileptic seizures would likely occur in the context of discussing her past traumatic experience in therapy. Because Helen was intelligent and resilient, I expected she would work hard in therapy. I anticipated she might have trouble if she ever felt she had not lived up to my expectations, since she grew up believing that if she did not live up to her family's expectations she would be rejected. She also frequently asked me for advice or my opinion, and I anticipated that I would feel pulled to maintain her in a dependent position.

As a new therapist, I knew that I was going to be vulnerable to the strong countertransference reactions involved in treating patients with trauma. Specifically, I had a feeling of being a guilty bystander and not doing enough to help her.

COURSE OF TREATMENT

Initially, the treatment involved education about PTSD and its symptoms. Helen was relieved to know that her symptoms had a name and had been experienced by other people as well. We discussed various options for PTSD treatment and decided to proceed with prolonged exposure, a manualized therapy. prolonged exposure (PE) is a behaviorally based therapy that aims to reduce the emotional intensity of flashbacks through confronting the disturbing memories in a controlled fashion. It also develops improved coping skills through exposures to reduce avoidance.

I initially encouraged Helen to undertake this type of therapy because I conceptualized her main issue as PTSD. I had a supervisor who was certified in PE so I had been discussing this form of therapy a great deal in supervision. As a psychotherapist in training, PE appealed to me because it was manualized. I was intimidated by treating someone with extensive childhood sexual abuse. I felt that the outline from the manual would be something I could cling to for support while I was navigating through sessions alone with Helen.

Not long into treatment, however, it became apparent that Helen's case was not amenable to a highly structured approach. Her deafness limited our ability to record the sessions so she could listen to them later, which is a major therapeutic component of the PE technique. Furthermore, Helen had tremendous difficulty discussing her traumatic experiences. She would stutter and spend long periods silently reexperiencing the traumatic situation with eyes either closed or staring. Despite frequent encouragement, she was initially unable to put these experiences into more than staccato phrases. This made it difficult to retell the memory multiple times, which is another key therapeutic component of PE.

After a few sessions, my PE supervisor suggested that I stop PE and switch to a psychodynamic approach. My supervisor was concerned that Helen was not in a safe situation where she felt removed from her trauma. Helen entered therapy living in an apartment frequented by substance-abusing male friends of her roommate. She later left that situation but returned home to live with the perpetrator of her early sexual abuse (though she said no abuse was currently taking place). One of the requirements of PE is that the participant be in a secure environment in order to be able to tolerate intensive discussion of past trauma.

I discussed Helen's living situation with her. She said she understood the issues but did not have the financial means to live on her own. Helen said the structure of the sessions did not matter to her. What she found helpful in therapy was the freedom to talk about "forbidden" things. Helen told me that her mother told her that she was angry with her for seeing a therapist and discussing family "secrets." But, she felt so much better after bringing these secrets to light that she was willing to defy her mother and continue in therapy.

With both my supervisor and Helen encouraging the switch, I had to confront my own issues about exchanging a highly structured therapy for one that had no checklists. At that point, I had gained some experience with discussing difficult topics so I felt less anxious about proceeding without a manual in front of me.

Shortly after starting treatment with me, Helen was admitted for video electroencephalogram monitoring to evaluate her seizures. Helen had to stay in the hospital until she had a shaking episode that could be studied. Because her hospital stay lasted several days, I agreed to visit her for a brief session in the hospital. When I arrived she appeared dysphoric. She told me she had had a shaking episode on the unit. The neurologist had just told her that they were able to determine that the episode was a nonepileptic psychogenic seizure. Helen said she understood the neurologist's explanation that when she was shaking there were no epileptic patterns on the monitor. She confided that she felt ashamed that her seizures were not "real."

As in times past, Helen drew on her natural courage and intelligence to deal with this new diagnosis. When I saw her at the next visit in my office she said she had accepted the diagnosis of psychogenic nonepileptic seizures (PNS). She had agreed with the neurologist that she no longer needed to see him or take antiepileptic drugs. She reported that she wanted to understand these episodes and work hard in therapy so she could return to work. With the support of Helen's neurologist, we were able to move forward to address these episodes as part of the disassociation and somatization phenomena that are often adaptations to trauma.

As soon as we began to discuss her previous trauma, Helen began having nonepileptic seizures in the office. These episodes began with stuttering and staring which progressed to shaking of her arms, legs, and head. The first time one of these episodes occurred was anxiety-provoking, even though I knew they were likely to happen. I sat there debating whether I needed to go for help and whether I could leave Helen alone while I did so. As the shaking continued, I tried talking to Helen to bring her out of it but she did not respond. As I sat there trying to think of what would get her attention, I remembered that she was a soccer fan. In my drawer I had a photo of my kids in their soccer uniforms. I held the photo in front of Helen and told her to look at the photos. That did eventually cause her to focus on the present, and she stopped shaking. I wanted to process this in supervision because I was uncomfortable with my disclosure. Although Helen asked me about my children a few times after that, we were able to move on and leave the issue of my family behind. I believe Helen enjoyed discussing my family because it made our interaction more personal and informal. However, I felt shifting attention to my personal life was another form of resistance that shifted attention away from the hard work of identifying and expressing Helen's own feelings.

My supervisor challenged me to bring up the issue of these shaking episodes in session. It felt awkward to me, but I mentioned to Helen that the shaking episodes interfered with treatment by limiting our interaction together. I suggested that we develop a plan to bring her back to awareness when an episode occurred. Helen did not appear uncomfortable with the topic, but she also did not have much to say in response. I suggested that I would call her name or tell her to pet her guide dog if she had brought him to the session as ways to get her attention. Her only comment was that she agreed that she did not want me to touch her to get her attention, because that would make her feel like her personal space had been violated.

At this stage in therapy, Helen frequently ended sessions by saying she did not see how therapy was helping her. As she would leave I struggled with guilt. I was the one who had encouraged Helen to enter therapy at the neurology clinic. I assured her that if she was willing to cross the divide from treating her problem in a medical clinic to treating it in a psychiatric clinic it would get better. When she told me that she did not feel better I felt that I had let her down. I gave in to her resistance and did not push her to talk about uncomfortable topics; effectively, I allowed her to control the sessions. When I discussed this in supervision and saw where I had enacted this countertransference, I resolved to and go back the next week to try again. However, despite my best intentions, I continued to find that when I looked back at the end of a session, I had not found a way to move the therapy forward. This happened over and over again.

The penultimate hindrance to therapy came when Helen became completely deaf. This occurred precipitously when she developed a perforated eardrum from an infection. She was devastated because she could no longer carry things off as if she could hear. Her whole life had been focused on functioning as if she could hear in order to maintain acceptance from her family and friends. As time wore on, the possibility that her hearing was permanently gone loomed large. The process of discussing her past trauma was pushed into the background by the need to discuss her feelings about the loss of hearing and her fears that her family would abandon her because they had already made it clear that they could not cope with her hearing impairment.

I had initially expected her to be able to continue to read my lips. However, after several attempts with her shaking her head in frustration and saying that she did not understand, I grabbed some paper and started writing out my questions, which she would then answer. This was a challenging new twist for a novice therapist. I already struggled with formulating questions appropriately, and now I had to figure out how to distill each question into a few jotted words on paper. It was also physically tiring to do so much writing. I felt worn out after each session.

Written on paper, my words and meaning were not distorted by hearing impairment. I immediately noticed that our dialogue was more focused. I felt humbled when I realized that Helen had only been pretending to understand much of what I had been saying before. I thought we were connecting and making therapeutic progress when, in fact, Helen had been left behind while I relentlessly pressed forward. Helen apologized profusely for the way her hearing impairment now inconvenienced me. She brought me presents of tablets and pens (which I thanked her for but refused). Gradually I realized that I had been involved in an enactment. When I had been carrying on as if she had almost no hearing impairment, I was acting in the family role of pretending that the hearing impairment was a nonissue. To Helen, I was someone else who needed to be kept happy and not inconvenienced by the extra demands of deafness. When I drew attention to these patterns, Helen agreed with the interpretation but continued to focus on my comfort rather than her own needs.

A defining moment came when she began to see me as different from her family. At the end of a session, Helen expressed her concern that my hand must be cramped from all the writing I had to do to communicate with her. She also said how afraid she was that she would remain deaf. Without much thought except to end the session and move on to the next patient, I wrote, "It doesn't matter to me if you stay deaf. We can still do therapy." Suddenly, her face broke into a bright smile. I was taken aback because I had become so used to her flat emotional persona. "Really?" she said. I wrote, "Sure." She said how glad she was because she liked therapy. She left the session with a palpable sense of relief. It was an emotionally charged experience for me, and I was glad to be able to discuss it in supervision later that day. I was unprepared for how a simple almost off-handed comment by me could elicit such a strong reaction in a patient. Instead of abandonment she felt acceptance, and it was profound for her and me.

Helen was also very accepting of me as an inexperienced therapist.

At this point in therapy we had the awkward experience of leaving the session by different routes but ending up sitting across from each other on the same commuter train. I had not discussed a plan for how we would react when we saw each other in public. I thought it proper that a therapist should ignore the patient so as not to draw attention to our relationship in public. However, I also knew that Helen was hearing impaired. While I took the train regularly, Helen did not. I knew she had inadvertently sat in the wrong section. Not only would she not be able to hear the announcer when it was time for her stop, but when she saw the train pull up she might not have enough time to get to the front of the train to the necessary exit door. Would it empower Helen for me to tell her to move forward? Or would it foster dependence? After a few seconds, I decided that for better or for worse I needed to intervene. So I leaned across the aisle and indicated that she should move to the front car. To my chagrin, I could tell from her reaction that she felt rejected. She thought I was communicating that I did not want to sit by her and that she should be the one to move! I explained again that only certain train doors would open at her stop and I was concerned that she would not make it in time if she remained in the present car. She then smiled appreciatively and got up and moved. I discussed this episode in supervision and then later with Helen in the next session. We ended up laughing about it, and the therapeutic alliance was not damaged. We agreed that if we crossed paths at the train station again, we would not acknowledge each other.

Then the day came when Helen's fear became a reality. Helen reported in her typical emotionally detached way that the specialist had finally determined that her hearing was permanently and completely impaired. She talked about how she could not cry. She was numb and afraid that her family and friends would abandon her. I tried to help her put her feelings into words. I asked her to talk about the things she would miss now that she had lost all hearing. She talked about missing the sound of TV, the car radio and music, the bark of her dog, and then she added, "And your voice." I was deeply touched. Once again, I observed the power of our relationship. I felt an overwhelming sadness, and I struggled with the tears that she could not cry. That day I developed a deeper appreciation of the power of projective identification. I didn't cry, but I sure wanted to.

Now that the deafness was permanent, Helen agreed to try doing therapy with an ASL interpreter. This introduced an interesting dynamic into the therapy. The interpreters were always women, but we were not able to have the same one each time. Helen was resilient enough to tolerate this variability in who was present each week. The content of our discussions at this time revolved around Helen's struggles with her new identity as a deaf person. She felt cut off from the hearing world. However, she believed the deaf world would reject her because she communicated orally. I observed her to have transference reactions to the interpreter. She would look to her for approval and acceptance as if she represented the deaf world. I was self-conscious trying to figure out how to do therapy in front of an audience. At times I would look to the interpreter for approval when I was discussing deaf culture! Despite being distracting and limiting, the interpreter helped the therapeutic alliance by demonstrating in a concrete way that I accepted Helen as a deaf person.

With Helen's deafness, we had to discuss how to handle the nonepileptic seizures. I could no longer call her name to bring her out of an episode. I felt out of control especially when she was disassociated and shaking and I had to sit there watching with an interpreter beside me. My supervisor encouraged me to discuss this at the beginning of the next session. Helen said she was not comfortable with me touching her with my hand, so we decided that I would lightly tap her leg with a tissue box to get her attention.

At this point, my supervisor and I discussed how to deal with advice about managing her medical issues. Because she was getting advice from so many others, I felt that giving advice would increase the transferential issues related to her need to please. In order to help Helen identify and express her own beliefs and feelings, I felt it was important to remain neutral about this advice. Helen was torn about whether she should have a cochlear implant to restore some of her hearing. Her family was pressuring her to have the procedure.

We had discussed Helen's issues with cochlear implants even before her ear infection. Helen had said she did not want an implant due to the artificial nature of the sound and the risks of surgery. Personally, I felt rushing to get the implant at this time was another way of trying to please her family and protect against abandonment. My feelings of anger toward her family for rejecting her based on her deafness colored my attitude toward getting the implant to please them. However, it was important for Helen to make the decision herself. We discussed the risks of the procedure not working and the fact that the new sounds would not be like the natural sounds she previously was able to hear. Helen was focused on feeling that she would be accepted again as a full member of the family if she was able to get enough hearing to function in the hearing world. In the end, she decided to get the implant.

One day while we were discussing the implant, she unexpectedly had a nonepileptic seizure in the session. This was the first time a nonepileptic seizure occurred when discussing something other than her past trauma. As we processed what had just happened in this new context, we were able to determine that the episode occurred because Helen felt fear about the upcoming surgical procedure. This was the first time Helen was able to recognize and label the emotion of fear in herself. Previously, when I had asked Helen to describe how she was feeling prior to the onset of a shaking spell, she would only say "restless." As we discussed the past episodes compared with the current one, Helen realized that these shaking episodes were a reaction to fear. She said that this understanding helped her feel more in control. Now Helen had a word to express how she was feeling. I hoped that by bringing clarity to her inner conflict she would now be able to process it on a conscious level.

Just as we had that breakthrough in therapy, we had to stop our sessions for about 3 months due to her surgery. During her recovery she would text me occasionally to report how she was doing. She appeared to enjoy being cared for by her parents. She reported that her father was especially kind to her while she was recovering.

She finally was able to make an appointment for therapy. At that visit she discussed how she found the implant much harder to adjust to than she thought it was going to be. The sound quality was mechanical and strange. Also her brain had not readapted to filtering out the background noise. She heard everything and it was exhausting. Her family had begun to lose patience with her, expecting that she should be back to "normal." She reported that she spent most of her day secluded in her room. I was not able to provide much supportive therapy as Helen could not tolerate more than 20 to 30 minutes in session.

Eventually, with the help of speech therapy, Helen was able to tolerate the sounds from the implant. However, she started coming to each session using a cane. She reported that she had developed left-sided weakness that no one had been able to explain. The cane made her feel vulnerable as she navigated the train station, and eventually she began using a walker. Helen went to several neurologists who told her there was no structural cause for the weakness. At one point she brought me the records to review. I told her I also did not see evidence of a neurological reason for the weakness. I believed this weakness was a new unconscious way of expressing her inner conflict about her relationship with her family. It also provided reasons for Helen to remain in the sick role and receive sympathy and support from her family.

Eventually, she came to session and said that she went to a neurologist who told her that he felt she had had a stroke from the implant too small to be detected by tests. While she felt satisfied that this explained her weakness, she talked about how she struggled with hearing the word "stroke." She was upset to think that she was so young to have something that happened to "old people."

This new development tried my patience as a novice therapist. I had trouble setting aside my background as a medical doctor to enter into her world. It made me angry to spend 50 minutes discussing her stroke when I was convinced that she had not had a vascular event. While she had been open to discuss the fact that her seizures were not medically explained, I sensed she was not willing to give up the idea that she had had a stroke. While in the past a neurologist had "shamed" her by looking at a test and saying that her seizures were nonepileptic, she now had found a new neurologist who was willing to set aside test results and agree with her belief that her body had been damaged. While I was not sure if it was on a conscious or unconscious level, I felt that Helen very much wanted to remain dependent on others through the security of the sick role, which now focused around her unexplained leg weakness. She had a familiar purpose in life (i.e., seeing multiple doctors) and could avoid returning to the unpleasant task of addressing her past trauma.

Although I was not conscious of it at the time, I experienced this as a narcissistic injury. In the split between the "good" neurologist who believed her and the "bad" neurologist who "shamed" her, I aligned with the "bad" neurologist. I felt anger toward the "good" neurologist who I felt was practicing sloppy medicine. From this point on, I felt disconnected from Helen. At the time I thought it was Helen who had closed herself off emotionally due to the trauma of surgery. I can now see that part of the distance was my anger that she had rejected my opinion as to the cause of her weakness and chosen to assume the sick role again.

Therapy now revolved around the continuing conflict for Helen between the desire to be cared for versus the desire to be independent. She no longer talked about leaving her parent's home. She now experienced life behind the protective embrace of her metal walker. She would react to others encouraging her on by walking more slowly and becoming more exaggerated in her unsteady gait. One mistake I would make during this phase was to get frustrated with her slow progress down the hall toward my office. It was a manifestation of my deeper anger that I believed she had rejected my help and decided to "give up." Although I tried to mask my irritation, I am sure she noticed and that contributed to the emotional distance between us.

From a psychodynamic perspective, it is likely that Helen's prior traumatic experiences predisposed her to having difficulty coping with having an implant. Like other trauma survivors, she was sensitive to compromise of her body integrity. She coped by regressing to her previous coping style—forming her identity about a somatic illness. Previously it was nonepileptic seizures; now it was unexplained leg weakness. This weakness also kept her in the familiar position of being dependent, passive, fearful, and powerless. At a time when she could view life as a new beginning with her newfound hearing, she redefined her identity post-implant as that of a person at the end stage of life without hope for improvement. She responded with indifference when the physical therapist discharged her because she was not making progress. She appeared content with the new pattern of relating to the world from behind a walker festooned with a homemade cloth carry bag like one would see in a nursing home.

TERMINATION

Before I had fully recognized and processed these new countertransference reactions, it was time to begin the termination phase of our treatment. It was not an ideal time to separate, but the date was fast approaching when I would graduate and leave the clinic. We discussed our mutual feelings of sadness that our time working together was coming to a close. Our interaction became more superficial and she no longer had nonepileptic seizures in the office. Helen exhibited her characteristic resilience when she agreed to take on the emotionally difficult process of transferring to another resident for continued psychotherapy.

Throughout this termination period, Helen often cancelled appointments. We only met a few more times before graduation. These visits were stilted and she seemed emotionally distant. When I tried to explore her feelings of anger toward me for leaving, she strongly denied them. I felt frustrated that she was not engaged. There was an undercurrent of anger in the room. I felt guilty that she had to terminate under such circumstances.

ASSESSMENT OF PROGRESS

Through supervision, I was able to come to a balanced understanding of Helen's progress. Over the 2 years that we worked together, Helen had transitioned from someone naïve to treatment to someone who understood and accepted the benefits of psychotherapy. She found comfort in understanding the diagnosis of PTSD. She was willing to address the PTSD symptoms through symptom-focused cognitive-behavioral therapy and then was willing to switch to dynamic psychotherapy when it became clear that there were too many hindrances to effective cognitive-behavioral therapy. Through dynamic therapy she was able to experience emotional understanding and connectedness through a therapeutic relationship that was different from relationships in her past. She shared very personal and intense experiences and found that she was not rejected. She experienced complete hearing loss and the therapeutic relationship continued on. She expressed anger toward her parents in session and there were no consequences. She realized the value in having a place to express and experience life issues therapeutically.

During our therapeutic interaction, Helen was able to accept the diagnosis that her episodes were nonepileptic. This was a large paradigm shift since she had believed that they were seizures for about 7 years. The diagnosis enabled her to stop antiepileptic medications and return to driving. It also provided a stimulus for her to engage in the work of therapy to understand these episodes.

When Helen was finally able to identify feelings of fear as the stimulus for her episodes, she began the deeper process of learning to identify and express her feelings. One of the most disturbing things for Helen was that her emotional numbness blocked both positive and negative feelings. She said that she watched others reacting but she could not feel. By the end of our treatment, she was better able to clarify that when she felt "restless," it was either fear or anger. She was also able to experience and express positive feelings toward me when she felt accepted.

Helen benefited overall from having her experience clarified as PTSD. She expressed that it was helpful to know, for example, that her frequent nightmares were part of the syndrome and that others have similar experiences as well. She still required medication to help her sleep at night. However, when she woke up with paralyzing fear, she did not feel so alone.

Helen also said it was helpful to explore her deaf identify in therapy. The ASL interpreter who could align with her in explaining deaf culture to me helped as well. In our sessions, she was able to experiment with manual communication without feeling judged by either family or the anti-oral part of the deaf community. As Steinberg (1991) writes in her article on treating hearing-impaired persons, "Working with deaf clients may be the ultimate challenge for mental health professionals, requiring them to explore the nature of the relationship between thought and language and between the communication of thought and the development of a personal identity" (p. 380). We were able to help Helen forge an identity as someone who perceives the world and expresses her thoughts differently from her hearing family.

Helen's communication was also influenced by her past trauma. When she first came to treatment, she spent long periods of time sitting without speaking. She was so overwhelmed with speaking about things she had spent her life suppressing that she could not find words. As therapy progressed, she was better able to put her thoughts into words, either verbally or through signing to the interpreter. When we reached termination phase, Helen was able to say that she thought therapy was helpful. She wanted to continue the process with another therapist.

As a novice therapist, I entered treatment with Helen expecting to rescue her from her suffering from untreated trauma following a quick checklist. This experience taught me to have more realistic expectations about the pace of therapy. When we started, we were able to quickly define the core problem. At times, therapy progressed according to plan but at other times our progress would plateau. Helen engaged in multiple types of resistance including everything from nonepileptic seizures and periods of silence to bringing her guide dog and focusing on him throughout the session. It was helpful to study typical countertransferences and technique issues through reading and supervision to keep our sessions directed toward the core problem.

I now understand that the technique of psychodynamic psychotherapy is a road map but the journey is different for each clinical dyad. When I consider therapeutic goals for therapy for the core problem of trauma, I see that Helen has already benefited from therapy. She has developed enough trust to be able to transfer from one therapist to another. She was empowered to be able to determine the plan for how the transition would take place. She benefited from the mutual respect that we shared. She expressed a sense of security in being free to be deaf in the therapeutic milieu. She was also empowered by being able to determine for herself that the nonepileptic seizures were her way of expressing fear.

The vignette about the experience that Helen and I had on the commuter train is a metaphor of the journey Helen and I took in therapy. Our paths randomly crossed in a neurology clinic in the same way that we happened to sit next to each other on the train. I understood the theory about what a therapist should do upon encountering a patient in public just like I understood the theory of how to approach problem-focused psychotherapy. However, I struggled with how to apply the theory, and in both situations, Helen's hearing impairment was a factor that influenced the pace and outcome of our interactions. It led to misunderstandings and miscommunication. But accepting and working with her hearing impairment also led to a deeper therapeutic alliance through trust. We traveled together for a time and then parted ways. We both have been enriched by the journey.

REFERENCES

Nowak, D., & Fink, G. (2009). Psychogenic movement disorders: Aetiology, phenomenology, neuroanatomical correlates and therapeutic approaches. *NeuroImage, 47,* 1015–1025.

Steinberg, A. (1991). Issues in providing mental health services to hearing-impaired persons. *Hospital and Community Psychiatry, 42*(4), 380–388.

CHAPTER 14

SLAYING THE DRAGON

A Case of Trauma

MARGOT MONTGOMERY O'DONNELL

Mark is a young man with serious poly-substance abuse, including heroin addiction, who underwent a multimodality treatment involving inpatient rehabilitation, maintenance therapy with Suboxone (a newer and better version of methadone), addiction counseling, and individual psychotherapy. The therapist describes carefully how psychodynamic therapy contributed to his recovery and the relevance of a newly recognized childhood trauma as a predisposing factor in his addiction.

The case history details three intense instances of therapeutic engagement, illustrating how weeks of work can come together in moments of powerful self-awareness for the patient and increased closeness between therapist and patient. The patient becomes more open to remembering important events of his child-hood, and this leads the way to a better understanding of his reaction to those events and their subsequent effect on him and his substance abuse. Although the patient will likely continue to be vulnerable to relapse of his addiction, his self-awareness, confidence, and function are markedly increased with the treatment. This successful therapy culminates in a dream that encapsulates the patient's problem and his continuing struggles with anger and addiction.

CHIEF COMPLAINT AND PRESENTATION

Mark presented to the outpatient dual diagnosis resident clinic at the beginning of his senior year at a nearby university. He was a tall, slightly unkempt young man who smelled strongly of cigarette smoke. At his first visit, he reported that he was in recovery from an assortment of substances and that his drug of choice was heroin. He was being treated for opiate dependence by a psychiatrist in his hometown with Suboxone (buprenorphine/naloxone) and was seeking weekly psychotherapy because his psychiatrist required it in order to prescribe Suboxone maintenance. The clinic where I work was close to his school.*

Mark was honest and open discussing his addiction history. He reported drinking alcohol in eighth grade and smoking marijuana in high school. During his last year of high school, he began spending time with an older group of friends who used and sold hard drugs. He experimented with methamphetamine and cocaine, including crack cocaine, and used heroin both intranasally and intravenously. Three years ago, he participated in an intensive outpatient treatment program which resulted in almost 9 months of sobriety. He relapsed when opiates were prescribed for a surgical procedure, and his addiction quickly escalated thereafter. With the support of his family, he enrolled in outpatient opiate maintenance treatment with Suboxone near his home. He had several relapses early in treatment but eventually achieved 9 months of sobriety from heroin by taking this medication and by attending monthly medication management appointments and recovery-based group therapy.

In our first session, Mark said he was seeking treatment primarily in order to continue receiving his Suboxone treatment. However, he went on to describe feeling anxious much of the time. He felt short of breath inexplicably and worried about physical ailments. At the start of his sixth year of college, he was disappointed with his academic performance. He believed he was capable of completing the work he was assigned, but always seemed to run out of time and miss deadlines. He described a conscious conflict between feeling significantly older than his peers, yet less well equipped for the upcoming events: graduation, employment, and close relationships. He worried aloud that he was "broken."

HISTORY

Mark was the only child of working class parents. His father was the second-generation owner/operator of a family construction company

---

* Suboxone (buprenorphine/naloxone) is an opiod receptor partial agonist that is approved for the treatment of opiate dependence. It must be prescribed by a physician in an office-based practice with special training and certification by the Drug Enforcement Agency. Suboxone, like methadone, is often called replacement or maintenance therapy because the buprenorphine replaces previous illicit opiates and dramatically improves the chances of maintaining sobriety.

founded by Mark's paternal grandfather. His mother worked for a florist before becoming a homemaker. He described his dad as a "guys' guy" who did not show much affection, though Mark happily recalled sitting on his dad's lap learning guitar and driving the company truck. He begrudgingly acknowledged that his father drank frequently and threw "temper tantrums," but strongly denied physical abuse. He found his mother to be kind and "always there for everybody." Mark was very firm that his parents were "nothing but supportive." However, as early as the first session, he explained how he and his mother carefully edited the information they told his father about his addiction.

Mark's developmental history was notable for his premature birth. "I was so small that I fit in my mom's hands." Mark initially denied any history of trauma but did share the following story. When Mark was first born, his parents were young and struggling financially. As his father worked to learn the family business, he saved up money, and instead of moving to a nicer apartment, he began building a "dream home." Mark remembers moving into the "giant house" just before starting first grade. One day, only a few months after moving in, his mother was staining wood in the garage. She left the rags unattended while she picked Mark up from school. When they drove home, the road was full of fire engines and police cars. His father was on the lawn with moderate burn injuries. The house burned almost completely to the ground.

Mark saw very little significance in this event and only shared it when prompted. He reported his father wanted to "move forward" and seldom spoke of the loss. Mark and his parents moved back into his paternal grandparents' home and then into a trailer parked on the property as they rebuilt. His father drank more during these years and did not spend as much time with the family. Mark understood his father was busy but also worried he was angry and blamed him and his mother for the fire. They did not move back into the new home until Mark was in third grade. It was at about this age that Mark started feeling uncomfortable and anxious around classmates and neighborhood friends. He remembers feeling confused about this and describes feeling like he was "different" and did not belong. "It was like I was this laidback happy kid one day, and then suddenly couldn't do anything right or easy. Everybody else had life figured out and I had missed something."

Mark's happiest memories revolved around soccer and music. He recalled, fondly and warmly, learning to play his father's guitar. For high school, Mark transitioned from his small school in a working middle class neighborhood to a large township high school. He recalls being struck by his sense of "outsider-ness" and social anxiety. He felt embarrassed to raise his hand in class and did not make many friends. He did not try out for the soccer team because of an ankle injury, but also because he was uncomfortable about taking criticism from the coaches and feared being cut from the team.

Mark drank alcohol and smoked marijuana through junior year. He had average academic performance and spent most of his time playing music in his parent's basement with his best friend. During his senior year, Mark made friends with an older group of teens already deep into the hard drug culture. Mark tried methamphetamine, cocaine, and heroin and admits that being high alleviated much of his chronic anxiety and self-consciousness. Though he applied late, Mark was admitted to a local university with a good reputation in the creative arts. The summer after high school graduation, he underwent a painful surgery for his deviated septum, a condition he had suffered since childhood. He quickly destroyed the reconstruction with intranasal cocaine use.

Once at college, Mark barely passed his first semester and made few new friends. During Christmas break, he met his first "real" girlfriend. She attended a boarding high school near his home and they regularly spent time together on the weekends. Early on, Mark found her emotions erratic and difficult to predict; she would occasionally cut herself to relieve stress. But he was drawn to "protecting her" and often drove from his school in the middle of the night to "save" her from a party when she had had too much to drink and blacked out. When she was sober, she was a perfectionist and worked for hours every day on her studies.

Mark used drugs regularly and heavily during his second year of college. He failed the majority of his classes and, by the summer after his sophomore year, he was "unraveling." He revealed his addiction to his girlfriend who helped him tell his mother. He enrolled in and completed a 3-month intensive outpatient addiction program over the summer and was allowed to restart school in the fall. After a scheduled repair of his previous septum surgery, Mark misused his prescription pain medication by supplementing with street opiates. At the end of his third year in college, he was fighting over the phone with his girlfriend, and she began to threaten suicide. She hung up the phone and, several hours later, a mutual friend called Mark to say that his girlfriend was in the emergency room following an overdose. Mark got in the car to race to the hospital but "ended up" purchasing and using heroin.

Mark's addiction escalated to daily heroin use for several months. He told his mother about his use, and she helped him find and enroll in a Suboxone treatment program near his home where regular group and individual addiction counseling were required in order to receive the medication. He initially continued to use heroin sporadically. He described his mother as very supportive, both financially and emotionally.

However, he reports that the two of them were careful not to reveal the full extent of his addiction to his father. "Pills are ok, but if my dad knew about the needles he'd lose his s---." He completed 9 months of regular treatment before seeking psychotherapy.

CORE PSYCHODYNAMIC PROBLEM AND FORMULATION

Part I: Summarizing Statement

Mark is a 24-year-old white male in his sixth and senior year at a local university. He has a history of poly-substance dependence, including cocaine and heroin, and is currently on opiate maintenance treatment. Mark struggles to identify his strengths and what is important to him, as he spent so much time and energy in his past absorbed by drug use. He complains of episodes of panic with shortness of breath and he currently has few friends. He has difficulty completing academic work on time and often turns in assignments late or incomplete. He has had one serious romantic relationship with an unstable woman who abused alcohol. A massive house fire at age 6 was traumatic, though Mark describes it as having little impact on his life and expresses almost no emotion when describing the event.

Part II: Description of Nondynamic Factors

Mark meets DSM-5 criteria for substance dependence in remission (marijuana, cocaine, methamphetamine) and opiate dependence in remission on maintenance therapy, as well as subthreshold anxiety. He describes his mother as "anxious" though she has never been diagnosed or treated. Both of his parents drink alcohol regularly, and he has a maternal uncle and paternal cousin with severe drug and alcohol addictions, so there is likely genetic risk for addiction on both sides of the family.

Mark reports hard drug use since 18 years old, with alcohol and marijuana experimentation prior to that. His longest previous period of sobriety was 9 months as a result of intensive outpatient rehabilitation. Currently, he has been sober for almost that long with opiate replacement therapy. His sustained drug use in adolescence and young adulthood may have affected his brain maturation and the development of neural regions specific to reward and mood. Mark was prescribed quetiapine (Seroquel) during his first outpatient treatment, which was helpful for sleep but did not improve his anxiety or sense of "outsiderness." He did not continue it after leaving the program and has not taken any other psychiatric medications.

Part III: Psychodynamic Explanation of Central Conflicts

Clearly, Mark's biggest problem is his addiction, but Summers and Barber (2010) do not identify addiction as a core psychodynamic problem. The contemporary conceptualization of addiction involves genetic vulnerability along with psychosocial risk factors. One of these risk factors is trauma, and from a psychodynamic perspective, Mark is struggling with the core problem of trauma.

Though Mark does not identify a violent trauma, such as assault or combat, I believe that when his home burned down, he lost his basic sense of trust in the world and in his parents' ability to keep him safe. He responded to the trauma with numbness and avoidance, growing anxious at school and seeking to minimize these frightening feelings with distraction and eventually drugs. Any feeling of anger or disappointment about his father's lack of involvement was avoided, as was any awareness of conflict between his parents.

Mark felt close to his mother and secretly guilty because of this. Though he respected and admired his father, he feared his father's disapproval and disappointment, and shared his secrets with his mother, only increasing his feeling of guilt. Mark's traumatic experience made him feel different from others. He managed this painful feeling of differentness and guilt by abusing substances. He spent years of addiction avoiding his feelings with intoxicants and now feels numb even when he is not under the influence. He experiences panic with physical anxiety symptoms like shortness of breath and occasional stomach upset, often without a clear trigger.

When Mark met his girlfriend, he enjoyed protecting her from other men and from herself. This made him feel big and powerful, and in charge of events, rather than a victim of them. He was reenacting the traumatic scenario with the house, by trying to save his girlfriend like he wanted to save his mother and father from their loss. He fantasized that he could control threatening situations in hopes of keeping himself and his family safe. But, despite his best efforts, his girlfriend continued to put herself in increasingly dangerous positions, and this constant threat triggered Mark's feeling that the world is unsafe and untrustworthy.

According to Summers and Barber (2010), "common secondary effects of trauma include a disturbance in identity . . . [and] avoidance." Mark believes he is a talented musician who generally cares about people in his life, but he does not know who he is or how he will move forward. He is crippled in school by the inability to complete assignments on time due to a pattern of perfectionism, which delays his creative process. He avoids anxiety regarding upcoming deadlines by playing videogames or, previously in his life, by using intoxicants.

The psychodynamic and biological factors in Mark's life affect one another. His opiate and dopamine systems, both integral to reward and attachment, were likely affected by repeated substance use during important periods of maturation. This series of insults to those systems may have led to an increased vulnerability to anxiety and uncertainty. During Mark's addiction, he was often in unpredictable and dangerous situations with other addicts and dealers. Thus, his participation in the drug culture resulted in repetitions of trauma, including witnessing assaults, overdoses, and experiencing arrests. Mark's strengths include creative talents and a love of learning.

Part IV: Predicting Responses to the Therapeutic Situation

Mark was fascinated by the neurobiology of anxiety and addiction, and he started psychotherapy with a lot of excitement, hoping to use biological and psychological theories to understand himself better. He was sober and motivated for change. Mark greatly disliked the Twelve Step approach to sobriety, but enjoyed learning about and integrating the biological information about addiction that had been introduced in his first outpatient treatment. He experienced two significant periods of sobriety since developing his dependence and previous sobriety is a strong predictor of extended recovery. However, he has always had difficulty connecting to treatment providers and trusting authority figures, probably because he saw his father as a strict and rigid childhood authority figure, as well as his fear of reprisal for rule breaking.

Mark missed several appointments with his current addiction counselor because he wanted to avoid being "scolded" for not attending Twelve Step meetings. But he only succeeded in delaying and magnifying the consequences as the coordinating doctor decreased his Suboxone dose in response to his noncompliance.

In the current treatment, Mark may idealize me as the treating therapist while acting out in ways that jeopardize his treatment. He will likely vacillate between accepting and rejecting trauma as an explanatory narrative for his current difficulties. He may feel protected by me since I am a female therapist, just as he felt protected by his mother from his father's disappointment and anger. In this regard, he may look to recreate the collusion that he shares with his mother. At other times, he may hide his behaviors from me as he does from his father, since I am an authority figure. He may try to impress me with his talent, insight, and good behavior, as he often hoped to impress his girlfriend, to gain love and secure attachment.

Mark has already had significant benefit from opiate replacement therapy. The strong legal and ethical boundaries required for Suboxone treatment may provide safety and consistency early in treatment, as providers must be specially licensed and patients sign contracts agreeing to weekly therapy, urine drug tests, or pill counts. However, the increase in expectations provides a clear opportunity for Mark to self-sabotage.

COURSE OF TREATMENT

Early attempts at establishing a traditional therapeutic alliance were halting and heavily influenced by the necessity of establishing boundaries. After only one therapy session, it seemed to me there would be potential therapeutic benefits to Mark, and clear educational benefits for me, to integrating his care by having me serve as both his pharmacotherapist and his psychotherapist. Coming from a split care model, Mark needed several sessions to warm up to the new relationship between his therapy and the responsible use of his prescriptions. At the initiation of therapy, Mark was fairly disorganized and needed support for keeping a calendar and remembering appointments.

Two months into treatment, he lost a paper prescription and missed a session in the same week. What he perceived as a "weird coincidence," I interpreted as significant risk behavior. As a trainee, I was keenly afraid of being naïve or manipulated by the patient. On one hand, I feared Mark was lying about the prescription to get extra pills to sell or abuse, which made me feel like a "sucker." On the other hand, I worried he had relapsed and did not want to face the appointment, which made me feel like a failure. Supervision was helpful in calming my insecurities and helping me focus on the patient's needs. For example, I could confirm with the pharmacy and his insurance company regarding his most recent prescription and any attempts to double-fill. Of course, there are ways to circumvent this monitoring, but it provided me some assurance.

The standard of care for Suboxone treatment requires regular drug testing. In addiction treatment, only observed urine drug screens are considered reliable. All other methods are fairly easy to manipulate and the temptation to do so is prominent for some patients. But while urine drug screening calmed my fear of being manipulated, it caused different anxieties about physical boundaries. I already found the regular blood pressure and physical exams for signs of opiate withdrawal uncomfortable in the psychotherapy relationship, and Mark behaved differently in the exam room, which was down the hall from my office, than he did in sessions. He was uncharacteristically jovial and silly, which I experienced as flirtatious. I shared my feelings in supervision and discussed how, early in treatment, stricter boundaries would likely serve Mark better than an awkward and uncomfortable exploration of the transference. So Mark completed his urine drug screens at an outside facility, and the clinic nurse monitored his vital signs for indications of opiate withdrawal whenever we decreased his medication dose.

I used supervision liberally throughout Mark's treatment to handle the medical and dynamic challenges of his case. I worried about the establishment of a traditional therapeutic relationship while prescribing powerful medication that required strict behavioral controls. I finally began to relax after 6 months of treatment. That week, Mark called the office, which was unusual. On the phone, he told me that the pharmacy had made a mistake in filling his monthly prescription, dispensing four times his prescribed dose! After the lost prescription incident, we had talked about the importance of transparency around his medications. We decided together that he should take the medication back to the pharmacy and make them aware of the error. Unfortunately, the pharmacy could not reissue the correct dosage without charging for a second prescription, which would entail a dramatic out-of-pocket expense for Mark. After discussion, my supervisor agreed to hold the prescription in our clinic according to approved storage procedures. Mark brought the full prescription to us that same day, and I dispensed his medication from the office for 4 months. This transparency on Mark's part, and the degree of control on my part, made it easier for me to trust him.

To illustrate the changes Mark made during therapy, I will review three important clinical moments. They show Mark's work at increasing insight, identifying and managing his anxiety, improving organizational skills, and expanding his emotional range to include more joy as well as anger.

The first significant moment in therapy exemplifies Mark's improved ability to deal more directly with his procrastination and sense of foreshortened future (a typical sequel of trauma). Mark's early session content mostly centered on his anxiety and poor performance in school. As it was his senior year, Mark was required to complete a project. He also needed to complete a full load of required courses that he had previously failed or not completed. Mark had a pretty accurate sense of his abilities but was disorganized. He started projects and classes with great motivation and high expectations, but got distracted or "bored" or "accidentally" missed assignments. He often offered the following excuses for missed assignments: "I overslept," "I was playing videogames," and "I didn't remember the assignment." Inevitably, he would find himself at the end of the semester with more work than he could conceivably accomplish. He rushed to complete the projects and was generally disappointed with the results.

We explored these work habits, which had begun in elementary school at about the same time as his anxiety. I wondered aloud if, like his parents working so hard for the house only to have it burn down, he did not trust that his hard work would produce a good outcome. Instead he always expected the proverbial rug to be pulled out from under him. Such a mindset, I mused aloud, would make it hard to choose schoolwork, with its comparatively long-term outcome, over playing video games, with their short-term rewards. Mark was silent for a few moments before agreeing that this was, at least, a strange coincidence. "Yeah," he said, "I've never thought I would live very long or have much of a future. That's weird to think about it connected to the house." Mark sat quietly for a few more minutes, and began to smile. "I guess it's also kind of like using [drugs]. When I was using, I couldn't think about the future at all . . . like consequences and stuff." We talked together about how sobriety allowed him to function better day-to-day. However, being "clean" was not his sole long-term goal and he needed to start planning for the future. Staying "clean" was necessary, but not sufficient, to take on his life developmental goals.

For several more sessions, Mark and I worked on the idea that trauma can cause a sense of a foreshortened future, and how this had contributed to his disorganization and procrastination. We reviewed some basic study and organizational skills he could use to be more prepared, and plan his time. Mark continued to procrastinate, but could now catch himself and redouble his efforts in certain areas. He often used session time to help structure his week and plan for assignments.

The second important clinical moment occurred after almost 9 months of therapy. Despite some continued inconsistency in his work, Mark was going to be eligible for graduation. His new habits were paying off. With reluctance, Mark began to talk about his plans for his future after graduation and about continuing treatment. He wanted to be off opiate maintenance at some point, but was ambivalent about the potential discomfort of withdrawal. He wanted to start a career in music but was "just getting the hang of school." He occasionally worked for his father for extra money, but could not imagine living at home and learning the family business.

At the time I was also transitioning from my third to fourth (and final) year of residency. This meant a change in schedule, a change in office space, and a new deadline looming—termination of therapy. Mark explored his confusion about how to support himself after graduation, but seemed unconcerned about the possibility of termination in another year. Together, we crafted a plan to decrease the Suboxone dose every 3 months, leaving 3 months of treatment available when Mark would be sober without any opiate maintenance. I expressed concern, echoed by my supervisors, that this timeline might not be long enough to ensure success. Mark would reassure me, "You know I do better with deadlines, Doc." This was a clear foreshadowing of events to come.

As the sessions developed a more future-oriented focus, Mark complained more about his health. He had gained significant weight since beginning treatment and felt out of shape. His work for school was mostly sedentary and he ate a typical college diet of pizza, hoagies, chicken wings, and cheesesteaks. He often presented out-of-breath from running up the two flights of stairs to my office.

He described other instances of feeling chest "tightness" and shortness of breath. At first, he could not describe when these events would occur. Eventually, he saw a pattern. They occurred mostly in class and when he worked on his senior project. I was suspicious of an anxiety component to Mark's pulmonary concerns, but considering his history of otolaryngology issues and status as a regular smoker, I encouraged him to seek medical care. Once he had a clear bill of health, and another doctor's recommendation to discontinue tobacco, I inquired whether Mark thought his breathing issues could represent anxiety. While he spent many sessions talking about his future plans, or lack thereof, he denied having "anything to be anxious about."

After a few sessions like this, however, Mark noticed out loud that his breathing was always better after psychotherapy. I commented, "You mean, talking takes a weight off your chest?" He liked the metaphor and agreed to consider that his body was physically expressing the stress and anxiety about the future that he had a hard time expressing any other way. As he shared more and more about his fears regarding the societal and personal expectations of adulthood and responsibility, his physical anxiety symptoms became more manageable and more predictable. I suspect that he worried equally about failing or succeeding after graduation, as failure would bring disappointment but success might bring challenges he could not handle. Therapy did not solve this conflict, but talking through multiple subtle variations of the theme released some of the internal paralysis and helped him feel more flexible, even "lighter."

The third important clinical moment happened when Mark identified avoidance in his relationships with others. We called this "using dirtiness as a defense." As he began imagining a real future for himself, he saw that he had few friends and minimal social connections. He had not been in a romantic relationship since his relapse. He spent many weekends at his parents' home but did not keep in touch with any childhood friends. He lived with several classmates in a house near campus, but they all drank alcohol and went out a lot. Recently, they were teasing and sometimes insulting Mark about his isolation and housekeeping habits. I had certainly observed him unshaven at times and in clothes that looked like they had been ironed on the bedroom floor, but I was not sure how much to attribute to normal college bachelor behavior. Finally, I asked Mark to describe, objectively, how bad things really were.

He reported that his room was piled so high with dirty laundry he could barely open the bedroom door. He sheepishly admitted there were days, if not weeks, of dirty dishes under his bed and full ashtrays "all over." His description surprised me, and I was not very good at hiding my disgust! I was embarrassed to admit to my supervisor how judgmental my expression must have seemed. Mark took quick notice and stopped short. After I had composed myself, I told Mark that his report did not make his room, or him, sound very appealing. I immediately further regretted my comments. I knew the interpretation I wanted to make, but I felt clumsy and unrefined. Finally, I suggested to Mark that his room sounded like a fortress designed to keep people at a distance. Maybe he even felt that way about his hygiene and the way he dressed. He shrugged again and the time was up. I spent all week mortified by my behavior and feeling I had made a major therapeutic error by spontaneously reacting and judging, rather than exploring and trying to understand.

The next week, a well-dressed, clean-shaven Mark walked into my office with a broad smile. He was even wearing cologne. I was prepared to apologize for my therapeutic missteps the week before but did not get a chance. "You were right, Doc," Mark said, "this therapy thing is crazy." When I smiled, clearly not getting the joke, he continued. "I thought about what you said, how my being gross was keeping people away. So I went home and cleaned my whole room, I mean really cleaned my room, and did all my laundry. And I cleaned the kitchen and made dinner for everybody in the house. Then my roommates were going to this party and I went along. And I met this awesome girl. It's like you said, I took down the wall and all these awesome things happened. I met this girl and we have so much in common. She knows all the people I know, I can't believe I've never met her before. And she's really smart and works in music and already has connections. She's been over a bunch, and we're dating."

As the therapy up to this point was primarily about sobriety, schoolwork, and anxiety, I infrequently discussed transference issues in supervision and avoided them altogether in sessions. My supervisor and I had discussed the likelihood of a blandly positive transference based mostly on my roles as "expert" and teacher. Once the session content shifted to romance, however, my supervisor aggressively challenged my assertion. In response to Mark's rapid changes she offered casually, "He wants to please you." Now it was my turn to play a reluctant student. I clung to the emotional safety of my neutral stance and was extremely anxious about discussing, let alone working through, the complications of erotic transference. Finally, my supervisor laid it all out. She said, "Oh, of course there's erotic transference—there always is—men and women, old and young. It doesn't matter. You don't have to talk about it, especially since it's working well, but you have to admit to yourself that it's there." I agreed that Mark was making excellent progress in areas that mattered to him. I reluctantly accepted that erotic transference might be contributing to his motivation. I understood that my own discomfort was something to be explored in another setting. Mostly I was overwhelmingly relieved she did not expect me to offer interpretations about it.

After his transformation, Mark spent much more time discussing his relationships. He was the first member of his family to graduate from college, which led to discussions about family expectations and models of success. He loved and respected his grandfather, who had served in the military and started the family business. We discussed whether Mark would ever want to take over. He hated the idea, but had trouble explaining why.

He quickly realized that his new girlfriend was an alcoholic. Like his first girlfriend, she was smart and driven. She worked incessantly during the week, but would binge drink and blackout on weekends. She had a history with cocaine, but was not using anymore. She also had a history of rape while intoxicated only a few months before she and Mark met. Mark felt fiercely protective of her and committed to helping her become sober. While AA and NA meetings made him too socially anxious to tolerate, he could see how they would work perfectly for her. In the beginning of the relationship, she got sober for several months.

Mark became concerned about the relationship when his girlfriend returned to school after summer break. She struggled to maintain her sobriety and he began feeling depressed about not having much to do during the day. She was from a wealthy family, and Mark felt self-conscious about only working part-time for his family and in unpaid internships since graduation. She tried to hide her drinking at first, but eventually started coming home and picking mean, drunken, and sometimes violent fights. Mark got more and more depressed about this, though he never blamed her for the fighting and always "understood" the next day and accepted her apologies. He reported in several sessions that he "never" felt angry but often "just kind of numb" after fighting with her. He always felt relief when she cried and apologized. I encouraged him to explore how this was like his previous relationship, and we found many similarities but minimal insight into the bigger pattern.

I felt stuck during these sessions in a way I had not experienced before with Mark. I was slightly annoyed, even angry with him. I had not been angry when I thought he was abusing his medication or when he showed up late or risked failing a class. But now I was frustrated with his inability to stand up for himself and with my inability to help. Then, one day, he presented looking vulnerable and sad.

Mark and his girlfriend had been staying at his parents' house for the weekend. There was an accident at his father's work, and though no one was harmed, his dad came home red in the face and screaming. He yelled at Mark and at Mark's mom. He drank several beers very quickly and, after more yelling, went outside to drink in the garage. Mark's girlfriend was so upset that she went upstairs and stayed there for the day. When I asked Mark how he had felt, he said he felt "numb." I felt terrible for Mark, but I was also relieved and saw this incident as an opportunity to advance Mark's treatment. I always suspected that there was more trauma in Mark's childhood than just the fire. I thought perhaps his father was angry or violent in some way, but Mark always diverted discussions about his childhood. I assumed that he was not ready or that the frame of time-limited therapy was too fragile to handle his emotions. Now I could make an interpretation about his father's behavior in the present. I asked Mark if he felt the same kind of numbness with his father that he did with his girlfriend. He just nodded. He had already made the connection, and we both sat for several minutes in silence. We both knew it was time to talk about how much harder it was growing up in his house than he had initially wanted to admit—to me or to himself.

In the next session, I asked Mark how it felt to see his father act as he had when he was younger. It had been terrifying and he had started pretending it was not happening at all. He assured me there were only "a few" blowups that he could remember as a kid. Usually his father "came home from work exhausted and had a few beers and didn't yell at anybody." He never hit him or his mother. "After the fire he was always working so hard. He didn't have fun anymore. All I ever saw was my dad working hard, or my dad angry, or too exhausted to be angry." I wondered if somehow Mark blamed himself for the fire and also for his father's subsequent tirades.

We talked for several weeks about Mark's numbing response to seeing anger and his difficulty in letting himself feel angry. Mark said he would do almost anything to avoid feeling strong emotions, especially anger. I suggested that some of his anxiety might be about fear of feeling an emotion he could not control, and he agreed this was often the case. He pointed out that drugs had previously helped numb strong feelings, and we noted that his physical anxiety also helped neutralize emotional discomfort by converting it to somatic symptoms of chest tightness and trouble breathing.

Finally, we explored the connection between work and anger. Mark realized that he struggled to pick a career and was terrified of taking over the family business because he assumed that the only outcome of that kind of "success" was the unhappiness and anger he saw in his father. Now that he was sober, and a college graduate, he was paralyzed by his fear that a full, successful adult life meant tolerating all sorts of strong emotions, even anger. He had no idea how to do it.

As he explored more feelings about his childhood, Mark continued his romantic relationship. He and his girlfriend continued to fight and make up, and eventually she agreed to enter rehab. Mark did not fully understand his own behavior toward her. He thought he loved his girlfriend and might eventually marry her. But he did not know if this was a good enough reason to keep forgiving her. I pointed out that traumatized people may be drawn to repeat the experience, and perhaps his girlfriend's rage made him feel like his father used to.

Mark was uncomfortable facing the deeper implications of his father's traumatic anger and his own self-defeating behavior. So the next session I tried a different interpretation. I suggested that, in family systems, there is a balance of emotions and skills. For example, an under-responsible or chaotic parent will often raise an over-responsible and inhibited child to meet the family needs. Because his dad expressed so much anger and outward emotion, Mark kept quiet and tried to avoid his emotions. Then, since he had so little practice managing his emotions, he was afraid of his anger and uncomfortable in many social situations. This, I suggested, explained his attraction to women who were outwardly emotional, affectionate and dramatic. These kinds of relationships made him feel more in touch with his own emotions and more alive.

TERMINATION

As he approached the end of the second year of treatment, Mark had established a daily routine that met his immediate needs. He lived mostly with his parents and worked for his father several days of the week. In between, he stayed with his girlfriend and continued to make professional connections in the creative arts. He was taking a low dose of Suboxone daily and had been clean of illicit opiates for 3 years. The plan to complete the taper with 3 months of therapy still to go before my graduation had hit a snag. We slowed the taper over the winter to accommodate the difficult emotional work he was doing in exploring his childhood, and he had several missed sessions due to holiday scheduling and overtime at work. Now, we were scheduled to discontinue the medication and psychotherapy simultaneously. It was my turn to be anxious. I was concerned that Mark would lose two stabilizing factors at the same time, but he was enthusiastic. "It's better this way," he said. "I'm ready to really be on my own." Mark was also aware that I would be starting a small private practice after graduation and that he was welcome to continue treatment with me there, although it would cost him and his family considerably more than they had been paying for treatment so far. He could be assigned a new resident in the clinic for psychotherapy alone, or medication management, or both. He could find a therapist closer to home, as he now drove 70 minutes each way. Or he could attend Twelve Step meetings for support. Mark appreciated having options, but reminded me that he was, in his heart, a procrastinator and that he appreciated having a firm deadline. He wanted to graduate, as it were, along with me.

The session content shifted again to his future and his dreams. He was considering learning more about the bookkeeping side of his family's business and also wanted to consider joining the armed services. Working through his motivations challenged me to contain some of my own deeply held beliefs. I'm a proud member of a military family, and worked for the Veterans Affairs Medical Center after graduation. I believe military service is important to our country and beneficial for many individuals. But I also understand that service, especially in wartime, can cause terrible physical and psychological damage. Combat trauma increases the risk of substance use, posttraumatic stress disorder, depression, suicide, and relapse in those with a history of substance dependence. My instinct was to protect Mark from these dangers, but sharing this with him went against all our work about thinking for himself and challenging himself to move forward. His mother and girlfriend were understandably apprehensive, and it seemed best to explore their worries and fears, without introducing my own.

When Mark's Suboxone taper was complete and he was completely opiate-free, he had a dream. He was a knight with a shield and a sword. He was fighting a fire-breathing dragon chained to the entrance of a cave. He fought the dragon "with all [his] might" and pushed the dragon back into the cave before collapsing in relief. But the dragon would recover, and he would have to fight again. The dream seemed to go on like this forever. He always won, but the dragon never died. He was never exhausted, but always waiting to start another battle.

I encouraged Mark to free associate about different parts of the dream. The "world" in the dream was like a poster he had over the head of his bed as a child. He did not assign it any particular meaning and I noticed his resistance to exploring a clear reference to his childhood. He was suffering mild opiate withdrawal symptoms, and he wondered aloud if the dragon was like drugs—something he would have to fight all his life. I suggested to Mark that we are all the characters in our dreams, that part of him might be the dragon while another part is the knight. He thought the knight was the part of him that wanted to be a soldier and "fight for something bigger than myself, find some meaning in my life." I suggested the dragon might be his anger, which is also a part of him but which he does not really know how to handle fully. Neither of us commented on the presence of fire in the dream, though in retrospect it was the center of the dream and of the therapeutic work for almost 2 years. The dream seemed like a stunning summary of therapy. Mark understood that life would always be challenging and no longer wished to escape his situation or emotions with drugs or procrastination, with somatic symptoms or with emotional numbing.

ASSESSMENT OF PROGRESS

Mark was a thoroughly enjoyable patient to work with. He seldom missed appointments, though in the beginning I wondered how much that had to do with the efficacy of therapy and how much with the strict requirements for Suboxone treatment. My supervisor dragged me into acknowledging the role of transference in establishing and maintaining compliance and motivation for change.

Mark was usually open and honest. Even when he kept something back, he learned to watch himself and question his motives for such subversions. From the beginning, he thought psychotherapy was "cool" and always enjoyed interpretation and psychoeducation. He occasionally commented about the therapeutic relationship itself, expressing that he felt proud when I changed to a bigger office and wondering if he would be able to "sit in the other chair" when he "graduated."

Once he started dating, Mark worked hard to convince his girlfriend to seek regular psychotherapy. He complemented the work we were doing and imagined something like it would help her. "She has to stop drinking and start talking about her issues," he told me. "She can't do just one, it won't stick." He especially valued being able to talk about his old drug use and current medications in psychotherapy, using both psychological and biological explanations for feelings and behaviors.

Mark completed his Suboxone treatment 2 years after transferring his care to my clinic. He attended three additional sessions in my private practice. He continued to explore his interest in enlisting and discussed some of the real-world challenges it would present. He expressed pride and satisfaction about the progress of treatment, and believed he understood himself much better than when he started. He had acquired skills, not just for sobriety, but for adulthood.

In terms of symptoms, Mark never failed a drug test. I believe he took his medication mostly as prescribed with the intended results—craving management and lasting sobriety. His social anxiety was dramatically reduced and he seldom complained of pressure in his chest. When he did, he had a system for assessing his physical and emotional health to generate possible causes and interventions. Although he worried about a narrative "that just blames my parents," Mark found that his relationship with his father improved during the period he was discussing his childhood experiences. He understood his father's anger and explosiveness as a recurrent and chronic trauma in his childhood that was exacerbated by the house fire. He got better at telling when his father was open to conversation and using these times to talk about business and the future. He wanted to continue dating his girlfriend and was beginning to set reasonable boundaries on her behavior. He understood that if he enlisted he would not be around to help her and she would likely relapse.

Three months after completing treatment, Mark scheduled an additional appointment. He had been working closely with a recruitment officer and wanted to complete his enlistment packet. During the medical history and exam, he disclosed his opiate addiction and subsequent treatment. He needed a summary letter detailing his diagnosis, treatment, and prognosis in order to seek a waiver to enlist. After review of his file, I completed the letter and reviewed it with Mark. He again expressed his satisfaction with treatment and intent to stay sober and move forward with his life. I am unaware of whether he received his waiver and decided to enlist, but I wonder if I will see him again one day as a patient at the Veterans Affair Medical Center.

REFERENCES

Summers, R. F., & Barber, J. P. (2010). *Psychodynamic therapy: A guide to evidence-based practice.* New York: Guilford Press.

INDEX

An *f* following a page number indicates a figure; *t* following a page number indicates a table.

E

Eating disorders, 17*t*
Education. *See also* Psychoeducation
  clinical cases illustrating, 74–75
  core psychodynamic problem and, 17*t*
  depression and, 21
  therapeutic alliance and, 13
Ego psychology, 16*t*
Elicitation of feelings, 17*t*
Emotion regulation, 16*t*
Emotional exploration, 43–45
Empathy
  clinical cases illustrating, 132,
    184–185
  core psychodynamic problem and,
    17*t*, 18*t*
  fear of abandonment and, 28
  therapeutic alliance and, 13
  trauma and, 34
Empowerment
  core psychodynamic problem and, 18*t*
  trauma and, 34
Emptiness, 16*t*
Encouragement, 17*t*, 18*t*
Evaluation, 34
Expectations
  core psychodynamic problem and, 17*t*
  depression and, 20–21
Exploration, 34
Exploratory interventions, 18*t*
Exposure techniques, 232–233

F

Fear, 19*t*
Fear of abandonment. *See also* Core
    psychodynamic problem
  clinical cases illustrating, 139–156,
    157–174
  overview, 16*t*–19*t*, 25–28
Fear of being hurt, 16*t*
Feedback loop, 47
Feelings, 18*t*
Flexible attitude, 18*t*
Freedom
  core psychodynamic problem and, 19*t*
  obsessionality and, 25
Frequency of sessions, 17*t*
Frustration
  core psychodynamic problem and, 19*t*
  depression and, 20–21

obsessionality and, 25
termination and, 48
Futility, 19*t*

G

Genetic factors, 21
Goals of treatment. *See also* Therapeutic
    alliance
  change and, 43
  clinical cases illustrating, 75–76,
    89–90, 109, 111, 166, 171–172
  fear of abandonment and, 27
  low self-esteem and, 29
  overview, 11
  psychodynamic formulation and,
    39–40
  trauma and, 33
Grandiosity, 19*t*
Guilt
  clinical cases illustrating, 208–224
  core psychodynamic problem and,
    18*t*, 19*t*
  depression and, 20–23
  fear of abandonment and, 28

H

Helplessness
  core psychodynamic problem and, 19*t*
  fear of abandonment and, 28
Heuristic approach to diagnosis, 14–15.
    See also Diagnosis
Hope, 17*t*
Hopelessness, 18*t*
Hostility, 19*t*
Humanity, 17*t*
Hysterical character, 14. *See also* Core
    psychodynamic problem

I

Idealizing, 19*t*
Impulse control, 16*t*, 19*t*
Incompetency feelings, 19*t*
Inhibition, 32, 83
Insecure attachment, 25–26. *See also*
    Attachment
Intellectualization, 18*t*, 23
Intimacy, 16*t*
Isolation, 68–82
Isolation of affect, 18*t*, 23